the **About**.com guide to

GETTING
IN SHAPE

**Simple and Fun Exercises to Help
You Look and Feel Your Best!**

Paige Waehner, the About.com Guide to Exercise

Adams Media
Avon, Massachusetts

About About.com

About.com is a powerful network of 500 Guides—smart, passionate, accomplished people who are experts in their fields. About .com Guides live and work in more than twenty countries and celebrate their interests in thousands of topics. They have written books, appeared on national television programs, and won many vide the most interesting information for users, and for their passion for their subject and the Web. The selection process is rigorous—only 15 percent of those who apply actually become Guides. The following are some of the most important criteria by which they are chosen:

- High level of knowledge/passion for their topic
- Appropriate credentials
- Keen understanding of the Web experience
- Commitment to creating informative, actionable features

Each month more than 48 million people visit About.com. Whether you need home-repair and decorating ideas, recipes, movie trailers, or car-buying tips, About.com Guides can offer practical advice and solutions for everyday life. Wherever you land on About.com, you'll always find content that is relevant to your interests. If you're looking for "how to" advice on refinishing your deck, About.com will also show you the Tools You Need to get the job done. No matter where you are on About.com, or how you got there, you'll always find exactly what you're looking for!

About Your Guide

PAIGE WAEHNER is an ACE-certified personal trainer and freelance writer with more than twelve years of experience in fitness and exercise. She trains clients in their homes in the Chicago area, as well as online at PlusOneActive.com. She is the Exercise Guide at About.com, where she posts workouts, articles, and tips about exercise, and she has contributed to a variety of magazines such as *Desert Paradise* and *Pregnancy.* She is also the coauthor of *The Buzz on Exercise and Fitness* and author of the e-book *Guide to Be a Personal Fitness Trainer.*

Acknowledgments

Becoming a personal trainer and a writer have long been dreams of mine, and I wouldn't have made it without the help of my family and friends. I would like to thank my sister Kris for taking me through my first workout and teaching me the importance of having a strong, healthy body. I'd like to thank my husband, Adam, for supporting me throughout the many ups and downs of my ever-changing career, and Kim Hohman for being instrumental in helping me fulfill my dream to become a writer.

To my mother, Linda, and my sister Ashley: Thank you for inspiring me with your strength and support. Special thanks to my grandmother, Anna, for being the best role model for staying active I could ever have.

I would also like to thank the Health and Fitness Guides at About.com, who constantly inspire me with their creativity, intelligence, and insight into staying healthy and fit.

ABOUT.COM

CEO & President
Scott Meyer

COO
Andrew Pancer

SVP Content
Michael Daecher

Director, About Operations
Chris Murphy

Senior Web Designer
Jason Napolitano

ADAMS MEDIA

Editorial

Publishing Director
Gary M. Krebs

Managing Editor
Laura M. Daly

Acquisitions Editor
Brielle M. Kay

Development Editor
Katie McDonough

Marketing

Director of Marketing
Karen Cooper

Assistant Art Director
Frank Rivera

Production

Director of Manufacturing
Susan Beale

Associate Director of Production
Michelle Roy Kelly

Senior Book Designer
Colleen Cunningham

Published by Adams Media, an F+W Publications Company
57 Littlefield Street
Avon, MA 02322
www.adamsmedia.com

ISBN 10: 1-59869-278-X
ISBN 13: 978-1-59869-278-5

Printed in China.

J I H G F E D C B A

Library of Congress Cataloging-in-Publication Data is available from the publisher.

The exercise program within *The About.com Guide to Getting in Shape* or any other exercise program may result in injury. In light of the complex, individual, and specific nature of heath problems, consult your doctor before beginning this or any exercise program. If you begin to feel faint or dizzy while doing any of the exercises in this book, consult your doctor immediately.

This publication is designed to provide accurate and authoritative information with regard to the subject matter covered. It is sold with the understanding that the publisher is not engaged in rendering legal, accounting, or other professional advice. If legal advice or other expert assistance is required, the services of a competent professional person should be sought.
—From a *Declaration of Principles* jointly adopted by a Committee of the American Bar Association and a Committee of Publishers and Associations

Many of the designations used by manufacturers and sellers to distinguish their product are claimed as trademarks. Where those designations appear in this book and Adams Media was aware of a trademark claim, the designations have been printed with initial capital letters.

This book is available at quantity discounts for bulk purchases.
For information, please call 1-800-289-0963.

How to Use This Book

Each About.com book is written by an About.com Guide—an expert with experiential knowledge of his or her subject. While the book can stand on its own as a helpful resource, it can also be coupled with the corresponding About.com site for even more tips, tools, and advice. Each book will not only refer you back to About.com, but will also direct you to other useful Internet locations and print resources.

All About.com books include a special section at the end of each chapter called Get Linked. Here you'll find a few links back to the About.com site for even more great information on the topics discussed in that chapter. Depending on the topic, you could find links to such resources as photos, sheet music, quizzes, recipes, or product reviews.

About.com books also include four types of sidebars:

- **Ask Your Guide:** Detailed information in a question-and-answer format
- **Tools You Need:** Advice about researching, purchasing, and using a variety of tools for your projects
- **What's Hot:** All you need to know about the hottest trends and tips out there
- **Elsewhere on the Web:** References to other useful Internet locations

Each About.com book will take you on a personal tour of a certain topic, give you reliable advice, and leave you with the knowledge you need to achieve your goals.

CONTENTS

CONTENTS . . . *continued*

Introduction from Your Guide

Getting in shape isn't easy. In fact, for many people, the goal to get in shape and lose weight may be one of the most frustrating things they've ever tried to do. Why is it so hard? The answer to that question will be different depending on who you are, how you live, and what you want for yourself, but the simplest answer is this: It isn't hard if it's something you truly want. To believe that, you have to throw out a number of misconceptions about exercise and getting in shape, and in this book, I hope to help you do that.

At its most basic, getting in shape is about choices. When you make the choice to have water instead of soda or to walk up a flight of stairs instead of taking an elevator, you're getting in shape. When you choose to spend a few minutes of your day exercising instead of watching TV, you're getting in shape. If you make enough of these choices on a regular basis, you'll not only create new, healthier habits, but you'll also see changes in your body and your mind.

Obviously, it isn't easy making changes in how you live, but you're not alone. In this book, I'll help you understand what stops you from exercising so you can remove those obstacles in your path to create a healthier life. I'll help you set realistic, meaningful goals and create a specific plan to reach them so you can learn how to make those simple, healthy choices every day. I'll also help you learn the basics of exercise and the many different ways you can set up a program that fits your lifestyle, schedule, and goals.

By learning about how exercise works, the ins and outs of cardio exercise and flexibility training as well as the benefits and principles of strength training, you'll be able to create a simple program that gets you on the path to better health. The exercise section provides a list of basic moves for each muscle group, allowing you to work your entire body with whatever equipment you have available. The workout section provides a variety of workouts for every fitness level and every circumstance, whether you're just getting started or you're trying to figure out how to stay fit on the road.

In addition to understanding how your body works, you'll gain a deeper understanding of how your mind works, learning that even the smallest change can have a profound effect on how you feel and how you live. You'll understand more about the most elusive part of exercise: motivation. Many of us wait for motivation to come to us, as though we'll wake up one morning with a sudden desire to exercise. The truth is, motivation isn't something you wait for, it's something you create, and here you'll learn a variety of ways to do that.

The most important thing you'll learn in this book is that there is no right way to get in shape. The only right way is the way that works for you, and finding the right path is something all of us have to figure out on a daily basis. All it requires is a desire to change how you live and the willingness to move your body on a regular basis. A good dose of patience and a healthy sense of humor don't hurt, either.

Getting in shape doesn't have to be complicated, and it doesn't require that you change your life overnight. In fact, changing your life overnight is a sure way to overload your mind and body with too much change. But if you figure out where you want to be and keep your focus on where you are, you're already on the right track.

Chapter 1

Get Ready to Get in Shape

Preparing Your Mind for Exercise

When you think about getting in shape, what comes to mind? Maybe you think of how painful or boring it is, or maybe you feel guilty because you know you're not doing what you should do to be healthy and fit. The thought of exercise might bring up all kinds of negative feelings and thoughts that get in the way of your goal to get in shape. What do you do? Where do you start? How do you fit exercise into an already hectic schedule?

The good news is, exercise doesn't have to be confusing or painful, and even better, you don't have to feel guilty about where you are on the fitness continuum. The great thing about getting in shape is that anyone can do it, no matter what your fitness level is, how busy you are, or what your knowledge is about exercise. There's no "right" way to get in shape. The only right way is the way that works for you, and by taking things one step at a time as laid out in the following chapters, you'll be able to ease into an

About.

Exercise is so confusing. How do I know where to start?

▶ Don't panic! Getting started with exercise is simpler than you think, though it's easy to get confused with all the information out there. The best way to start is by keeping it simple. Don't try to do everything at once; instead, start with activities that are accessible and comfortable for you. Focus on establishing healthy exercise habits first, and slowly add more diverse activities over time.

exercise program that fits with your goals, your schedule, and the activities you enjoy.

Getting in shape starts with your mind, not your body. After all, it's your mind that usually gets in the way of your goals, isn't it? In fact, your mind may be working much harder than your body, coming up with all those great excuses for skipping your workouts (e.g., "I'd exercise, but I'm so tired and that sock drawer isn't going to organize itself …").

So, how do you retrain your mind to work with you instead of against you? The first step is to figure out what you really think about exercise. Whether this is your first attempt at exercise or your sixth, you already have preconceived notions about what it's going to feel like. These notions are based on your own experiences, what you hear and read in the media and what your friends and family say about their own experiences. Knowing what's behind your reluctance to exercise is crucial if you want to succeed at your goals.

These perceptions determine your choices, and if you think exercise is boring, painful, or confusing, how motivated will you be to do it? I don't know about you, but I want to spend as little time as possible being bored, in pain, and confused. The key is to examine those perceptions and change them so that exercise is something you want to do rather than something you have to do.

Get started by making a list of all the things you don't like about exercise. Be specific; don't just write "I hate exercise because it's boring," but explain exactly what's boring about it: "Exercise seems boring to me because when I walk on the treadmill, five minutes feels like five hours." Or rather than writing "I don't have time to exercise," you might write "Exercise takes time away from other tasks I think are more important."

Now, go back and examine your list and think of some solutions to those negative perceptions. How could you change your thinking or your program to make exercise more enjoyable? If the treadmill is boring to you, some solutions would be to try the elliptical trainer, walk outside with a friend, or try a workout video at home. If exercise seems less important than your other duties, one solution would be to ask yourself why your health is less important than other things in your life. Or perhaps you could look at your workout as the only time you have to yourself each day, your time to recharge and let your mind rest, with no phones, no errands, and no interruptions.

Now is your chance to look back on what you've been doing and see where you've gone wrong. It may be that you simply need to change your approach to exercise, choosing more activities you enjoy or creating a workout schedule that doesn't add more stress to your life. By exploring your feelings, perceptions, and preconceived notions, you can eliminate some of those negative thoughts that keep you from taking care of yourself. These thoughts won't go away overnight; it takes practice to change your thinking. But knowing what those thoughts are and where they come from will help you cultivate a more positive view of getting in shape.

Getting a Medical Clearance

Now that you've explored what's going on in your mind, it's time to focus on more practical steps to getting in shape. Starting an exercise program usually involves a variety of activities like cardio, strength-training exercises, and flexibility training. If you've never exercised or it's been a long time since you have, you might want to make an appointment with your doctor for a checkup to make sure you're ready to get started.

WHAT'S HOT

▶ I have a quiz called "Is Your Mind Ready for Exercise?" on my About.com site. It takes you through some simple questions to help you figure out what you think about exercise, and mistakes you might be making with your program. Do you do too much too soon? Do you have unrealistic expectations about what exercise can do for you? Bringing your perceptions to light is the first step toward changing them. Visit http://about.com/exercise/exercisequiz.

Not everyone will need a doctor's clearance to exercise, but if you've experienced any of the following situations, you might want to go ahead and make an appointment with your doctor before you get started:

- You have a family history of diabetes, heart disease, or other cardiovascular disease under the age of fifty-five
- You've been diagnosed with heart problems or have had heart surgery
- You have diabetes
- You're on medication for high blood pressure, heart disease, or diabetes
- You have any other medical conditions such as arthritis, osteoporosis, heart murmur, allergies, or asthma
- You experience pain or swelling in your joints
- You're pregnant or lactating
- You have problems with dizziness or fainting spells
- You're recovering from any type of injury or illness

It's especially important to talk to your doctor if you have any kind of joint problems; chronic injuries in the knees, hips, or shoulders; or if you have chronic lower back pain. There may be certain exercises or activities you should avoid, and your doctor may want to refer you to a physical therapist or other medical expert to help you heal any injuries.

You should also talk to your doctor about any medications you're taking. There are some medications that can affect your heart rate, such as calcium channel blockers (for high blood pressure or other heart problems), diuretics, and some asthma inhalers. If you're taking these types of medications, you may not be able to use your target heart rate zone to monitor your exercise intensity, and your doctor can offer other alternatives.

ELSEWHERE ON THE WEB

▶ When visiting your doctor for a checkup or to diagnose an injury, it's important to be prepared. About.com's Sports Medicine Guide provides some specific tips for getting the most out of your doctor visit in her article "How to Talk to Your Doctor." Just visit http://about.com/sportsmedicine/talktodoctor. You'll find suggestions for what to tell your doctor, what your doctor needs to know, and tips for making sure you have all the information you need to treat or manage your injury.

Proper Clothing and Footwear

Exercise clothes and shoes have come a long way in the past few decades. Just think of the shiny spandex phenomenon that swept the nation back in the 1980s and you'll probably agree that our choices now are at least more fashionable, if not more comfortable. These days, exercise clothes are more specialized—we have clothes for running, walking, aerobics, yoga, and cycling. Not only that, but there are a variety of high-tech fabrics to keep you warm and dry in the winter, cool and dry in the summer, and generally more comfortable all year round. Just walk into a sporting-goods store and you might be overwhelmed by rack after rack of high-tech, high-fashion clothes.

So, how do you know what clothes to get? The clothes you choose will depend on the workouts you're doing, your budget, and what you like. There aren't any special rules for what to wear, but you can use these general guidelines for stocking your fitness wardrobe:

- **Dress for comfort.** Choose clothes that won't chafe your skin, ride up, or shift when you least expect it. Wear what feels good to you, and you'll be more comfortable during workouts.
- **Choose clothes that fit your activity.** If you're a walker or runner, shorts and a T-shirt may work for you. If you're doing yoga, you may want to wear something more form fitting because baggy clothes can get in your way.
- **Choose quality clothes.** If you exercise more than a few times a week or you'll be outside in hot or cold weather, invest in sweat-wicking fabric like CoolMax. You'll be washing these clothes often, and quality clothes will last longer and keep you comfortable.

ELSEWHERE ON THE WEB

▶ Lower back pain is a common problem these days, and many experts think it's because we spend too much time sitting. It was once thought that resting was the best way to heal back pain, but research has found that exercise, specifically walking, helps patients recover faster. Wendy Bumgardner, the About.com Walking Guide, explains this in detail in her article "Walking Away Low Back Pain." Visit http://about .com/walking/lowbackpain.

- **Dress for the weather.** If you'll be outside in hot weather, dress in light-colored clothing to keep you cooler. When it's very cold, you'll want to dress in sweat-wicking layers to stay warm and dry.
- **Dress for safety.** If you're out at night, wear something reflective on your clothes and/or shoes so you don't get hit by a car. You may even want to wear a headlamp if there aren't streetlights nearby.

Updating your wardrobe should include paying attention to your athletic shoes. If you still have the same running shoes from ten years ago, it's time to spring for a new pair. But before you run out and buy any old shoe, it's important to choose the right shoe for the activities you'll be doing. If you plan on doing a variety of cardio and strength-training activities, you might try a cross-trainer. These are lightweight shoes designed to handle different activities for short periods of time.

But, if you're doing a specific activity several times a week, you'll want to invest in specialty shoes. If you're running, you'll need a good pair of running shoes that will fit your foot and running style. Visit a specialty running store in your area and bring your old shoes with you. The employees there will be experts at choosing the best shoe for your needs. If you're a walker, you can stick with walking shoes, which are stiffer and have less cushion than running shoes, although many walkers prefer running shoes because they're usually more comfortable.

Whatever shoe you choose, make sure:

- You have your feet measured, as foot size can change as you get older
- You try on the shoes with the socks you'll be wearing

WHAT'S HOT

▶ Buying workout clothes and gear online can save you time and money. Not only that, but you'll usually find much more variety at online stores than at your local sporting-goods store. Many online stores offer free shipping, discounts, and a flexible return/exchange policy, just in case something doesn't fit right. Just make sure the site you're visiting is reputable and one you trust.

- You shop at the end of the day; your feet swell throughout the day and you should try on shoes when your feet are at they're largest, to make sure they fit
- The shoes feel comfortable as soon as you try them on

Having the right pair of shoes can make a difference in how your workouts feel and can help keep you injury-free, so spend some time shopping around and trying on a variety of shoes. Don't feel that you have to buy the most expensive pair, although you should plan on spending anywhere from $50 to $100 depending on where you shop and what you buy.

Getting and Tracking Your Baseline Measurements

If your goal is to lose weight, gain weight, and/or change the shape of your body, one of the most important things you'll do is track your progress. The only way to know if you're going in the right direction is to know where you started. Are you losing fat? Gaining muscle? Improving your endurance and strength? Tracking a few basic numbers like weight, body measurements, and body fat percentage will ensure your body is making the right kinds of changes.

The most basic measurement to start with is your weight. If you tend to freak out about the number on the scale, just remember: A scale measures everything—bones, muscle, fat, organs, water, and what you've eaten. A scale won't tell you if you're losing fat or gaining muscle, so you'll need a few more measurements to monitor changes in your body composition.

Another basic number to keep track of is your body mass index (BMI). This is a calculation based on height and weight. BMI is a general way to see whether you fall into a healthy

▶ If you're a woman, the most important thing you'll need is a good sports bra. To choose the right one, start with brands that focus more on women's bodies, like Moving Comfort or Danskin. Most quality sports bras will have a Motion Control Rating (MCR) of low, medium, and high so you can determine the level of activity each bra can handle. Last, make sure the bra supports you without chafing or cutting off your circulation.

weight range, but like scale weight, this calculation does have some drawbacks. If you're very muscular or pregnant, your BMI may label you as overweight or obese even if you're not. The formula used to calculate BMI is:

BMI = (Your weight in pounds ÷ [Height in inches × Height in inches]) × 703

For example, if you weigh 165 pounds and are 65 inches tall, you would use the following calculations: $(165 \div [65 \times 65]) \times 703$ = 27.4 BMI

Use the following guidelines to determine how healthy your BMI is:

- **Obese:** Over 30
- **Overweight:** Between 25 and 29.9
- **Healthy:** Between 18.5 and 24.9
- **Underweight:** Below 18.5

Next up are your circumference measurements. Measuring different areas of your body is helpful in determining whether you're losing fat or muscle. Muscle is denser than fat, so if you gain muscle from your workouts, that could make the scale go up. But muscle also takes up less space than fat, which means your measurements will go down no matter what the scale says. It's best to measure as many areas as possible because we all lose body fat in a different order. At the very least, you'll want to measure around your chest, upper arm, forearm, waist, hips, thighs, and calves. Use the following guidelines when taking your measurements:

- Measure both arms and legs because most of us will find differences between the right and left sides of the body.
- For all areas except the waist, measure around the widest or largest part of each area; for the waist, measure around the smallest part or a half inch above the belly button.
- Hold the tape measure tight, but not so tight that it's digging into the skin.
- Don't "suck it in" while measuring.
- Wear the same clothes each time you measure yourself.

Tracking your body fat percentage is also helpful.   This will allow you to make sure you're losing fat and not muscle. There are a number of ways to test your body fat, some more accessible than others. The most accurate and the least accessible are hydrostatic weighing and DEXA (a kind of body scan), both of which have to be administered by medical and/or fitness professionals for a fee. Another option is to have your body fat measured by a fitness professional at a health club (if you're a member, many will do this for free). In this case, they might use calipers (fondly known as the "pinch test") to measure different areas of your body to calculate body fat. The accuracy of calipers largely depends on the tester, so you'll want an experienced pincher if you go this route.

Another option is bioelectrical impedance analysis, a technology used in body-fat scales. With these scales, an electrical signal is sent through the body (don't worry, you won't feel it), and your body fat is calculated based on how fast the signal moves (the faster it travels, the more muscle you have). This is the easiest method and, unfortunately, one of the least accurate because your results can vary wildly based on your hydration, skin temperature, and food intake.

ASK YOUR GUIDE

How often should I weigh myself?

▶ Weight fluctuates on a daily basis, so it's probably best to weigh yourself about once a week. Any more than that and you risk disappointment if the scale doesn't go down or, worse, goes up because of water weight gain or other factors. Be sure to weigh yourself at the same time each week as well— ideally in the morning before you've had any food or liquids.

Whichever test you choose, you can use the following table to get an idea of different categories of body fat for men and women:

BODY-FAT PERCENTAGES

Categories	Women	Men
Essential Fat	10–12%	2–4%
Athletes	14–20%	6–13%
Fitness	21–24%	14–17%
Acceptable	25–31%	18–25%
Obese	32% plus	25% plus

From the American Council on Exercise (ACE)

If you can't get your body fat tested, don't worry. The other measurements will work just fine.

Keep in mind that you don't have to track any of these measurements at all if you don't want to. Plenty of people use the very unscientific method of monitoring how their clothes fit. Most of us have a pair of pants or shorts that will instantly tell us whether we've gained or lost weight, and for some people, that's all they need to know. Do whatever works best for you.

Write it down. To make things easy, use the following form to record your weight, BMI, body fat, and measurements. Take your measurements every four weeks or so to see how you're doing. Try to avoid taking them every day or even every week, because these numbers don't show small, incremental changes your body is making, and that may discourage you, even though the changes are happening.

▶ If you're math phobic or just want to keep things simple, you might find online calculators helpful for getting some of your baseline measurements. My Body Mass Index (BMI) Calculator (http://about.com/exercise/bmicalc) does the work for you. Just plug in your weight in pounds and your height in inches; you'll get your BMI along with information about whether you're considered underweight, healthy, overweight, or obese.

PROGRESS CHART

Date: _____

Weight: _____

Height: _____

Body mass index (BMI): _____

Body fat: _____

Circumference Measurements:

Chest: _____

Upper arm (R/L): _____

Forearm (R/L): _____

Waist: _____

Hips: _____

Thigh (R/L): _____

Calves (R/L): _____

Recording your vital statistics and measurements is the first step in your journey to get in shape. But you'll also want to keep track of these numbers over time, and there are a variety of options for tracking your progress. One way is to simply use a form like the example above and make a note in your calendar or PDA to fill out a new form with new numbers every few weeks or so.

The Internet can come in handy here. If you like using a computer, have Internet access, and want more details about your progress, you might consider joining an online tracking Web site. Many of these Web sites offer free services that allow you to track everything from your weight and measurements to exercise and diet. What's nice about these kinds of sites is that there's nothing to download, and you can view a variety of charts, graphs, and

▶ The accuracy of body fat tests can vary widely depending on the test and the circumstances. Instead of focusing on that, look at that number as your starting place. As long as the number keeps going down, you'll know you're on the right track. If you're interested in exploring different ways to test your body fat, check out my article "What's Your Body Fat?" Just visit http://about.com/exercise/test bodyfat.

reports that show you exactly what progress you're making. Some sites offer different versions of their tracking software so you can choose free versions or more deluxe versions that offer more bells and whistles.

For example, FitWatch.com offers a free service that allows you to track your exercise, weight changes, and even your calories. The deluxe version, which has a subscription fee, has even more options, allowing you to set and track goals and create custom recipes. FitDay.com is another Web site that offers a free diet and weight-loss journal to track your progress.

Whatever method you choose, keeping track of where you are and how far you've come is just one way to stay motivated and make sure you're on the right track.

Overcoming Your Fear of Exercise

Taking practical steps toward getting in shape, like joining a gym or buying exercise equipment, can seem easy compared to actually doing the exercise. Most of us have fears when it comes to working out, and those fears can get in the way of reaching our goals. You might be afraid that exercise will hurt or that you'll make mistakes and look stupid in front of other people. You might be afraid you'll injure yourself by doing the wrong thing. Whatever your fears are, overcoming them is essential if you really want to get in shape.

If you're afraid exercise will hurt, try easing into a simple, basic program. For example, you might start out with three short walking workouts a week, with two basic strength-training workouts. Eventually, you'll want to work harder and longer, but by starting with a beginner program like the ones highlighted in Chapter 8, you can reduce or eliminate some of the pain you're anticipating. Delayed onset muscle soreness (DOMS) is something most of us have to deal with when trying a new activity, but easing into a program can help keep it at a minimum.

It's also important to know the difference between normal exercise sensations and genuine pain. It's normal to feel a burning in the muscles when you lift weights or a raised heart rate and respiration rate during cardio exercise. It isn't normal to feel shooting pains in your joints, connective tissue, or muscles, nor should you feel dizzy or lightheaded. These symptoms may mean you have an injury or other condition and should see your doctor if the pain doesn't go away within a few days.

If you're afraid to look silly or stupid, you're not alone. Anytime you do something you've never done before, you take the risk of making a mistake, and when it comes to exercise, many people think they should be good at it even if they've never done it before. And, keep in mind, anytime you have sweaty people swinging weights around, silly things are bound to happen. Visit any gym for a period of time and you're bound to see someone accidentally drop-kick his iPod, slide off the treadmill, drop a weight on their toe, or stumble during a kickboxing class.

If this worries you, one option is to stick with activities that are comfortable for you. You may not be ready to try that belly-dancing class at the gym, but walking on a treadmill may work just fine. Or if walking outside makes you feel self-conscious, you could try Leslie Sansone's *Walk Away the Pounds* videos at home. If you're at the gym, take advantage of the free orientation most clubs offer to learn how to use the machines, and don't be afraid to ask for help from the staff or even other exercisers. Most are happy to help, and you won't risk doing a push-up on the leg-press machine and wonder why it isn't working. Even better, find a friend or family member to go with you so you feel supported and less conspicuous.

ASK YOUR GUIDE

I feel intimidated at the gym. How can I feel more comfortable during my workouts?

▶ Walking into a gym can be intimidating, even for people who are in great shape and know what they're doing. To make the experience more comfortable, find a gym that has a welcoming atmosphere. You might need to find a smaller gym with fewer people and more support from the gym staff or a club that caters to just men or women.

Is it better to work out in the morning or in the evening?

▶ The best time to exercise is the time that works for you. There are some benefits to morning exercise; studies show that successful exercisers usually exercise in the morning, and exercise can make you feel more alert and energetic for the rest of the day. But if you're not a morning person, afternoon or evening exercise is just as good. A workout is a workout no matter when you do it.

Being afraid of getting injured is a healthy fear, but it shouldn't stop you from exercising. If you have an old injury or any other issues with your body, you may want to talk to your doctor, a physical therapist, or a personal trainer about what you should or shouldn't do. If you're healthy and there aren't any restrictions on what you can do, you can reduce your risk of injury by following a few basic rules:

- Always warm up before you exercise.
- Make sure you're wearing appropriate shoes.
- Use good form with all your exercises.
- Don't use so much weight that your form or posture suffers.
- Start with what your body is capable of and add intensity gradually.
- Stretch after your workout, paying close attention to any areas that are chronically tight, like the lower back or the hamstrings.

Another obstacle that often gets in the way of exercise is confusion. Walk into any gym and you'll find a sea of odd-shaped machines with cables and levers, all targeting different parts of the body. Where do you start? Walk into the fitness section of your local bookstore and you'll find shelves packed with books offering you the perfect exercise program. Which one is right for you? Turn on the TV and there are infomercials promising you instant weight loss in just minutes a day. Can that be true? Ask your friend how he lost so much weight and he might tell you he runs six miles a day. Do you really have to do *that*?

Knowing the right thing to do to reach your goals seems impossible with all the information out there, but it's important to know that there is no perfect exercise program. Any program can help you lose fat or get fit if you work hard at it, follow it consistently, and watch your calories. Clients often ask me, "What's the best cardio exercise?" My answer is always the same: the one you like the most. Yes, there are some activities that typically burn more calories than others. Running a mile in eight minutes will definitely burn more calories than taking a stroll for eight minutes, but if you hate running, how much time will you really spend doing it? Forget about what your friends say, and start with something you enjoy. The more you like it, the more you'll do it and the harder you'll work at it.

It's easy to get sidetracked with too much information. In fact, researching exercise can end up taking the place of actually doing something. Educating yourself is important, but at some point, you need to turn off the computer, stand up, and start moving your body. Don't worry about what to do ... in the next few chapters, you'll find tips and guidelines for setting up a balanced exercise program with ideas for cardio and strength-training exercises. So, rather than worry about whether you're choosing the right program, focus more on creating a balanced program you can live with on a day-to-day basis.

Finding Time

What's the number one reason given for skipping exercise? If you answered "not enough time," you get a gold star. Being too busy to exercise is a great excuse. Who can argue with a jam-packed schedule, right? On top of that, it's easy to use a busy schedule as a reason to skip workouts because there are no immediate consequences. If you miss a workout, it's not like you'll gain 10 pounds overnight (although some of us are convinced that really is possible), so it may not seem like a big deal. I hate to break it to you, but being too busy isn't the best excuse in the world. We now know that you don't have to have big chunks of time to get in shape. Researchers have found that splitting your workouts into three separate ten-minute workouts can be just as effective as doing thirty minutes of continuous exercise. You may have to plan ahead and be creative with your workouts if you don't have longer periods of time, but it can be done if you're really committed to getting in shape.

Some ideas for creative exercise might include walking the stairs at work on your break or using part of your lunch hour to walk around the neighborhood. Another idea might be to combine activities. I once had a client who would jog around the baseball field during his son's practice. I had another client who would put dinner in the oven and do an exercise video while waiting for it to cook. One busy client held walking meetings with his employees instead of sitting around a conference room.

It may take some time and effort to come up with unique ways to move your body, but it can be done. If you're having trouble fitting in exercise or knowing what to do with the time you have, you might consider working with an expert to help you figure out what you need to do. You'll learn all about finding a personal trainer in Chapter 2.

Get Linked

The following links to my About.com *Exercise site provide more resources for helping you get ready for exercise.*

YOU ARE WHAT YOU THINK

Negative thinking can come out in a variety of ways, especially when it comes to getting in shape. This article describes common patterns of behavior that can stand in the way of exercise. You'll also get some specific ideas for how to change those negative patterns.

 http://about.com/exercise/whatyouthink

EXERCISE EQUIPMENT AND APPAREL

If you like to shop online, check out this link. Here you'll find some of my favorite places to buy exercise clothes, shoes, and equipment. You'll also find reviews for a variety of products, including body-fat scales, fitness journals, and more.

 http://about.com/exercise/equipapparel

FINDING TIME TO EXERCISE

There are a number of reasons to skip workouts, from busy schedules to lack of motivation. But by making exercise a priority and learning how to make your workouts more fun, you'll find that fitting exercise into your life is easier than you think. This article offers basic tips for finding the time and motivation to exercise.

 http://about.com/exercise/findingtime

Chapter 1. Get Ready to Get in Shape | 17

The **ABOUT.com** *Guide to* **Getting in Shape**

Chapter 2

When, Where, and How to Exercise

Where Will You Exercise?

Your next step in your journey toward getting in shape is to choose where you want to exercise. Should you join a gym or exercise at home? One isn't necessarily better than the other, and they each have their own pros and cons, so your choice will be based on where you're most comfortable, what fits with your budget, and what you want out of your exercise program.

A home gym has its ups and downs. Working out at home can be a great choice if you don't have access to a gym, can't afford to join a gym, or just don't feel comfortable exercising in that kind of environment. There are a number of advantages to working out at home:

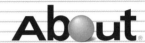

- **It's cheaper.** You don't have to pay membership fees, and you can create a home gym with very little equipment.
- **It's convenient.** You can work out anytime you like, wear what you want, and you never have to wait for the machines.
- **It saves time.** You don't have to pack a bag or drive to the gym, which can eat up a large part of your workout time.
- **It's private.** You can focus on your workouts instead of worrying about what other people are doing.
- **It allows for flexibility.** If your schedule changes, you can split your workouts or even squeeze in exercise while making dinner or watching TV.
- **It offers variety.** If you exercise at home, you can make your own workouts, follow workout videos, exercise outside, or even download streaming video workouts to your computer.

Of course, working out at home isn't for everyone. You'll need to be motivated and disciplined and enjoy working out by yourself. Some of the disadvantages of working out at home include:

- **There are distractions.** It's not hard to find reasons to skip your workouts if you exercise at home. Chores, family obligations, or your favorite TV show can become an excuse to skip your workouts.
- **It's easy to back off or quit.** Some people find they don't work as hard at home or they cut workouts short when they become difficult.
- **You might get bored.** Your home gym may not have the same choices a gym would have, so you may get bored using the same equipment time and time again.

- **You might not be very motivated.** If you prefer a more social environment, you may not be as motivated to do your workouts.
- **You might not know how to work out.** Working out at home may require some creativity, depending on the equipment you have and your knowledge of exercise.

Look through the two previous lists and ask yourself what you really want. Are you self-motivated and disciplined enough to do your workouts at home? Do you know how to set up a workout using the equipment you'll have? Do you need the energy of a gym to keep you going, or will you enjoy working out alone? Now let's look at the gym option.

Gyms have pluses and minuses.   You probably know a lot of people who go to the gym before or after work, or even on their lunch break. It's easy to see why gyms are so popular, as they definitely do have their advantages. Here are some examples:

- **It's an active environment.** Seeing other people working out all around you can be a great source of motivation. It's easy to find a person with a body you'd like to have, and it's also easy to find someone who's worse off than you are.
- **You can vary your workouts and enjoy some perks.** These days, gyms offer tons of bells and whistles, like pools and hot tubs, as well as lots of opportunity for varied workouts. You can join in on a kickboxing class, participate in a swimming workout, or even have a personal trainer guide you through your workout.
- **Many gyms offer child-care services.** Many gyms offer child-care services right in the building, making it easy for you to get a workout in without having to hire a babysitter.

WHAT'S HOT

▶ It's a great idea to check out a number of gyms online before you go visit them in person. Most large gym chains have Web sites with information about locations, costs, class offerings, hours, and more. Bally Total Fitness (www.ballytotalfitness.com) and Gold's Gym (www.golds gym.com) are two popular nationwide chains, and Curves (www.curves.com) is a gym just for women. Even if you don't end up choosing one of these gyms, you'll at least have a good idea of how much you can expect to pay and what you can expect to get out of your membership.

- **It's an opportunity to meet people.** Most people at a gym have something in common: They want to get or stay in shape. Though you're usually sweaty and a little out of breath, the gym is a great place to make friends and even find love!

Of course, gyms have some disadvantages, as well:

- **They can be expensive.** The cost of gym memberships just keeps climbing, with the low end being around $20 per month and the high end being around $80 per month. And don't forget about the initiation fee some gyms charge!
- **They can be crowded.** Gyms usually get crowded in the morning and then again in the evening when people get out of work. In addition to the likely possibility that a crowded gym will be hot and humid, you might also have to wait in line for a particular machine, sometimes doubling the time you spend at the gym without doubling your workout.
- **They run on a set schedule.** Most gyms have regular business hours, such as opening at 7:00 A.M. and closing at 9:00 P.M. But what if you're an early bird who likes to work out in the wee hours of the morning? And what if the aerobics class you want to take is only offered during the afternoon while you're at work?
- **You're on display.** People who are self-conscious about how they look or their low fitness level may feel uncomfortable working out in front of an audience. Though most people will be focused on their workouts and not on you, it can still be uncomfortable to sweat and pant in a public place.
- **You have to get there first.** Unless your gym is right down the street, you'll probably have to drive or take public transportation to get there. In inclement weather, you might find

it hard to force yourself to go all the way to the gym instead of just heading home after work.

Working Out at Home

If you've gone over all the pros and cons and feel comfortable working out at home, you're ready to set up your workout space. The equipment you choose will depend on your budget, how much space you have, and what your goals are. Before you buy any equipment, consider your exercise space. Will you have a separate exercise room, or will you have to work out in your living room or bedroom? Where will you store equipment like dumbbells, an exercise ball, or a barbell set? Another thing to consider is entertainment, especially if you'll be using a cardio machine. You'll want access to a TV or music so you don't get bored, so make sure that's available. Last, think about the environment. Will the room be cool enough in the summer? Warm enough in the winter? If you exercise indoors, there won't be any wind resistance to cool you off, so make sure you'll have a comfortable place to work out.

Start by thinking of what type of cardio equipment you might want. The most popular are treadmills, elliptical trainers, and stationary bikes, and the one you choose will be based on how much space you have, your budget, and the activities you enjoy.

The most popular is the treadmill, and the prices vary depending on whether you want a budget treadmill ($500–$1,500), a mid-range treadmill ($1,500–$3,000), or a high-quality treadmill ($3,000 and up). It's always best to get the highest-quality treadmill you can afford. A treadmill can be a significant investment, and the higher quality you get, the longer it will last. At the minimum, the American Council on Exercise recommends you choose one with

TOOLS YOU NEED

▶ If you're exercising at home, you might consider trying home exercise videos. You can find a variety of videos at places like Wal-Mart or Target, but many videos are sold through catalogs. Collage Video (www.collage video.com) offers a huge selection of exercise videos, as well as reviews of those videos, for every fitness level and every kind of workout you can imagine—from kickboxing and step aerobics to strength training and yoga.

a minimum 2.0 continuous-duty horsepower motor, a two-ply belt, and a sturdy frame that doesn't shake.

Elliptical trainers are also popular and may be a good choice if you'd like an activity that's low impact. Elliptical trainers range in price from $300 to $5,000, depending on the level of quality you choose. When buying an elliptical trainer, look for one that has a stride length of twenty-one inches, adjustable resistance and incline, and arm handles so you can work your upper body for a more intense workout. Make sure you measure how much space you have, especially ceiling height, and be sure to use the machine before you buy one. Some cheaper elliptical trainers can be loud enough to distract you during workouts.

Stationary bikes are another choice for home cardio exercise and might appeal to you if you need a gentle, no-impact workout. Stationary bikes range in price from $200 to $3,000, and like the other cardio machines mentioned, the price will be based on the quality and the extras (like programming or heart-rate monitor) included. When looking for a stationary bike, you'll need to choose between a recumbent (sitting with back support) or a standard upright model. The recumbent might be a good choice if you have any mobility problems or if you have a back injury, though you should always check with your doctor before doing any type of activity in that situation.

Another aspect in choosing stationary bikes is the type of resistance used. The cheaper models will use flywheels with a knob to adjust resistance, while others use air resistance generated by a fan in the wheel. Higher-quality bikes use magnetic resistance, which offers a smooth, quiet operation (cheaper bikes can be quite loud and need to be plugged in). Like any other machine you purchase, you want to make sure it's comfortable, fits in the space you have, and offers all the bells and whistles you need to keep you motivated.

ELSEWHERE ON THE WEB

▶ When buying a treadmill or any large piece of exercise equipment, make sure you do your research before you spend any money. Treadmill Doctor.com is an excellent resource, providing detailed information about what to look for in a treadmill. They also have a database of reviews covering all major treadmill brands and a Best Buy section that rates the best treadmills for your money.

Keep in mind that machines are not required to do cardio exercise. You can walk, run, or bike outside or create your own indoor workouts by doing things like jumping rope, jumping jacks, kickboxing moves, or even dancing. Chapter 4 discusses a variety of cardio activities that can be done at home, inside or outside, so don't feel that you have to run out and spend thousands of dollars on a machine you won't use.

Strength training is also an important part of your workout. The basic strength training equipment you might start with would include resistance tubes, dumbbells, and an exercise ball. Resistance tubes come in different levels of resistance (light, medium, and heavy), are cheap (usually less than $20 for a set of three), are versatile, and travel well. You can find resistance tubes at most sporting-goods stores and at discount stores like Wal-Mart and Target. If you don't have much space, are on a tight budget, or travel a lot, resistance tubes are a good choice.

Dumbbells are also great for strength training and can be used for all your major muscle groups. Eventually, you'll want a wide range of dumbbells (from 3 to 15 or more pounds) because some larger muscles will require more weight than will smaller muscles. But, if budget is an issue, you can always start with a few sets (from 3 to 8 or 10 pounds) and add on over time. Like everything else, dumbbells range from cheap (heavy-duty hex weights) to expensive (chrome weights), but unlike with larger purchases, going el cheapo on dumbbells isn't going to make much of a difference except for the look and comfort of the grip. You can find dumbbells at most major sporting-goods stores.

An exercise ball is also an excellent choice because it can be used in a variety of ways and usually costs less than $30. You can use it as a weight bench for upper-body exercises, a support for lower-body moves, for challenging ab work, and even as a chair

▶ Resistance bands are great tools for strength training because you can target every muscle in the body while having complete control over the resistance. But it's hard to know how to use them correctly. When you buy them, they'll usually come with a chart showing some basic exercises, but if you're looking for some workouts to try, check out my Strength Training with Resistance Bands Workout, which shows exercises targeting the upper body. Visit http:// about.com/exercise/bands workout.

▶ Adjustable weights are another option if you have space limitations and don't want dumbbells lying around the house. Adjustable dumbbells have all your weights included in one dumbbell and you simply turn a dial to release or add the weight you need for each exercise. Some can be very expensive (over $200) and bulky, but more recent versions are smaller and can end up being cheaper than buying several sets of dumbbells.

while you're working on the computer or watching TV. When choosing an exercise ball, make sure you get the right size for your height. A small, fifty-five-centimeter ball will fit a person up to five feet four inches tall; a medium, sixty-five-centimeter ball will fit a person from five feet five to five feet eleven inches tall; and a large, seventy-five-centimeter ball will fit a person who's six feet to six feet seven inches tall. You can find exercise balls at sporting-goods stores, discount stores like Target, and even in some bookstores.

If you want machine exercises that mimic the machines you'd find at a gym, you might purchase a multistation home gym. There are a variety of home gyms available, ranging anywhere from $500 to well over $5,000, and again, what you choose will be based on your budget, how much space you have, and what you want out of a home gym. Your best bet is to visit a variety of specialty fitness stores in your area to get a sense of what's available and what would work best for you and your family.

Before you buy large, expensive pieces of equipment, make sure you:

● Measure your exercise space, including ceiling height.
● Try machines before you buy them; plan on spending at least five minutes on each machine you're interested in, to make sure it's easy to use, fits your body, and has all the extras you want.
● Get the most for your money by choosing equipment that has multiple uses; for example, dumbbells are relatively inexpensive and can be used to work all your muscle groups, while something targeting just the abs or just the thighs may outlive its usefulness sooner than you think.

- Beware of buying products touted in infomercials; not all are bad, but many make false promises of fast weight loss with very little effort.
- Do your research. If you're buying a large piece of equipment, visit Epinions.com or subscribe to *Consumer Reports* for reviews about different types of exercise equipment.

Working Out at the Gym

While working out at home may sound appealing to some, the motivation and up-front cost it takes to get started might be too much for some people. Joining a gym is usually a quick and easy process, and you'll suddenly have a whole slew of equipment, classes, and trained staff available to you. While the money may not be so easy to let go of, the financial investment may motivate you to go on a regular basis. There's also a feeling of camaraderie and collective energy when you exercise at a gym that you don't get when working out by yourself. Of course, as you read in the first section, there are some disadvantages to gyms. In addition to high membership fees, you might have to deal with overcrowded workout areas and feeling uncomfortable working out in front of others.

The good news is that you have a variety of options for what type of gym you'd like to join. There are well-known chain health clubs like 24 Hour Fitness, Gold's Gym, Bally Total Fitness, and Life Time Fitness that offer cardio and strength-training equipment as well as fitness classes, personal training, basketball and racquetball courts, and, in some cases, indoor/outdoor swimming pools. Membership fees will vary depending on what club you're joining and where you live, but you should expect to pay some type of initiation fee (anywhere from $50 to over $300) and either sign a long-term contract or choose a month-to-month option. Joining a

TOOLS YOU NEED

▶ If you're on a tight budget, you don't have to spend a lot of money on exercise machines or gear. All you need is a little creativity and you can create your own weights with what you have around the house. My article "Exercising on the Cheap" will give you some ideas for making your own dumbbells and tips on where to find cheaper exercise equipment. Visit http://about.com/exercise/onthecheap.

chain is a good choice if you travel and can use your membership at clubs in different cities.

If you want a simpler approach, you can look in your local Yellow Pages for smaller, locally owned gyms or clubs that may offer cheaper memberships without all the bells and whistles. You can also find specialty gyms for bodybuilding, martial arts, boxing, yoga, or Pilates that may offer a variety of membership choices to fit your budget.

If environment is a factor, you may want to choose a women- or men-only health club. Curves is one option, a no-frills club offering thirty-minute circuit-training workouts with strength and cardio exercises for women. A new and growing trend is Cuts Fitness for Men, which involves the same type of circuit workout as Curves, but for men only. The downside of this type of club is that there are no other activities to try if you get bored or hit a plateau, so you may not want to get locked into a long-term contract.

Another option is your local YMCA or YWCA, which can be cost-effective and great for families since they offer a variety of family-friendly activities. Many towns and cities also have local community centers with fitness centers, pools, and classes for fees that may be cheaper than those at a larger health club.

Before you join a gym, you'll want to keep a few tips in mind:

- Make sure it's convenient to your office or your home and that it's open during the hours you want to exercise.
- Take a tour to make sure it has all the amenities you want and that it's clean and safe, especially the bathrooms. Check out the equipment to see if it's in good shape. If there are a lot of out-of-order signs, you may want to go elsewhere.

- Ask for a trial membership so you can visit the gym during the hours you'll be exercising, to see how crowded it is; try fitness classes and get a feel for the environment.
- If you'll be doing group fitness, check out the class schedule to see if the classes fit your schedule and needs.
- Don't be afraid to negotiate the initiation fee; some sales-people will reduce it or even waive it.
- Read the contract carefully; some gyms require you to sign up for a year or more and may have penalties if you cancel your membership during that time. Make sure the contract terms will work for you.

The Basics of Personal Training

If you're not sure where to start with exercise, one idea to consider is hiring a personal trainer. You don't necessarily need one, but a trainer can be a great resource if you're new to exercise, have injuries or physical issues, or if you need more accountability for sticking with your program. A personal trainer can offer:

- Motivation
- Accountability
- Customized programs to fit your schedule and goals
- Guidance for how to create efficient and effective workouts
- Education on which exercises to do and how to do them properly
- Expert help in reaching your fitness goals

A typical personal-training session costs anywhere from $25 to over $100, depending on where you live (if you live in a bigger city, fees will likely be higher) and the experience and education of your trainer. The average would most likely be between $50 and $100

▶ A personal trainer should help you with your exercise program and fitness goals. What she shouldn't do is diagnose injuries, give you meal plans to follow (unless she's a registered dietician or nutritionist), or give you exercises that cause pain or injury. If you're concerned that your trainer is crossing a line, my article "Choosing a Personal Trainer—Warning Flags" (http://about.com/ exercise/trainerredflags) can help you decide if it's time to fire your trainer.

for a typical hour-long personal-training session, and many trainers may have you sign up and prepay for a certain number of sessions at a time. If money is an issue, you can always discuss a payment plan with your trainer, or you can consider money-saving options like partner training (with a friend or family member) or half-hour sessions instead of a full hour.

When choosing a trainer, your best bet is to get a referral from a friend, family member, or someone you trust. If that isn't an option, you can find trainers at most major health clubs; personal-training studios; and even at some community centers, hospital fitness centers; or universities. If convenience is important to you, you might consider in-home personal training. Though it's usually more expensive because of the travel time, having a trainer come to your home might be a good choice if you have trouble sticking with your workouts, have a busy schedule, and want to work out in a comfortable environment. You don't necessarily need any equipment; many trainers will have portable equipment or they can advise you on the best equipment to get for home workouts. Just make sure you have some time without interruptions from work or family.

You can start your search in your local phone book or by using an online trainer-locater service such as UStrainersearch (www .ustrainersearch.com). If you're familiar with some of the personal-training certifications, you can also go to their Web sites to find trainers in your area. When choosing a trainer, you might want to interview several before deciding on whom to work with. At the very least, you want your trainer to have:

- A reputable personal-training certification (e.g., ACE, ACSM, NSCA, NASM, and AFAA are just a few well-known certifying organizations)
- A certification in CPR
- Liability insurance

- Experience, especially if you have special situations such as injuries or pregnancy
- A personality and training style that fit your needs

Beyond the basics, you should also make sure you feel comfortable with your trainer and that he listens to you, answers your questions, and gives you his full attention during sessions. If your relationship isn't working out for any reason, don't be afraid to talk to him about it. He may not be aware there's a problem. If things don't improve and you're not getting the most out of your sessions, move on to a new trainer.

Online Training

If working with a personal trainer is out of your budget or if you'd like some professional help without the face-to-face meetings, one recent trend is online personal training, or cyber-training. With this option, you typically pay a fee of anywhere from $9.95 to $39 a month to receive a workout program. Some sites offer ready-made workouts that are assigned to you based on your goals and fitness level, but if you want something more personal, you might choose a Web site that offers custom workouts created by your own personal trainer. In this case, you get all the benefits of working with a trainer but without the face-to-face sessions. You can communicate with your trainer through e-mail or on the phone, log your workouts, and get new workouts when needed.

When choosing an online trainer, you want to look for the same credentials as in a face-to-face trainer. The Web site should have trainers certified through well-known organizations, have experience with your goals, and should have a site that's easy to navigate. Look for sample workouts, exercises, or calendars if they're available, to make sure they're in a format you can understand and follow. Also, make sure they offer an exercise database with full descriptions and pictures of each exercise. Finally, avoid signing on with a trainer or Web site that pushes nutritional supplements or other questionable products, since, as mentioned previously, personal trainers shouldn't be giving you specific nutritional advice unless they have the education to do so. Once you find someone who has all the qualities you're looking for, you'll be ready to get started with a personal trainer!

Get Linked

The following resources on my 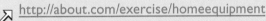 About.com *Exercise site provide more resources for helping you choose the right home fitness equipment, fit exercise into your schedule, and choose professionals to help you reach your goals.*

BEFORE YOU BUY HOME FITNESS EQUIPMENT

Before you spend a lot of money on home gym equipment, it's important to determine what you really need to reach your goals so you don't end up buying equipment you won't use. This article offers simple tips for choosing home fitness equipment to fit your budget, fitness goals, and available space.

 http://about.com/exercise/homeequipment

CHOOSING A PERSONAL TRAINER

Hiring a personal trainer can be a good move if you need help with setting up a workout program. Before you hire a trainer, you'll want a basic checklist for both choosing the right trainer and knowing when your relationship isn't working anymore. This article tells you what you need to know about hiring a personal trainer.

http://about.com/exercise/choosetrainer

ONLINE PERSONAL TRAINING RESOURCES

If you're interested in cyber-training and aren't sure where to start, visit my Online Personal Training index, which lists reviews of personal training Web sites as well as links to Web sites offering cyber-training. Many of these sites offer free trials or site tours, so take advantage of that and get a feel for the Web site and the workouts before you commit.

 http://about.com/exercise/onlinetraining

Chapter 3

Your Exercise Goals

Setting Realistic Goals

The single most important thing you'll do on your path to getting in shape will be setting your goals. It may seem like a no-brainer, but the goals you choose will set the tone for your entire exercise experience. Setting the wrong goal can be a determining factor in whether you exercise for a lifetime or for just a few weeks or months. The good news is, it's easy to set the right goals for you if you follow a few simple rules.

There are all kinds of ways to set exercise goals, but my favorite involves setting SMART goals. Normally, I'm not a big fan of acronyms, but I make an exception for the principles behind SMART goals:

- **S**pecific
- **M**easurable
- **A**ttainable
- **R**ealistic
- **T**ime oriented

Again, this may seem obvious, but many new exercisers make the mistake of setting goals that are too vague to measure, are impossible to reach, or have no deadline to keep them on track.

The confusing question is, what is a realistic goal? That's where things can get a bit fuzzy because there are no perfect goals—only goals that are perfect for you. As you're thinking of what you want to accomplish with your exercise program, look at each SMART element and ask yourself if your goals fit the bill.

Make goals specific. Too often, people set vague goals like wanting to tone up or exercise more each week. But what does toning up actually look like? And how much is more exercise? Get specific by figuring out exactly what you want to achieve. Instead of toning up, you might decide to drop a clothing size. Instead of deciding to exercise more, a specific goal would be to exercise at least three days a week.

Make goals measurable. Making your goal specific means you should also be able to measure it. Looking at the previous example, you can see that toning up isn't measurable, but dropping a clothing size is. Exercising more is hard to track, but deciding to exercise three days a week is a clearer goal that's easy to measure. Make sure the goals you set can be tracked and measured over time so you'll know if you're on the right path.

Make goals attainable. How often do you set impossible goals for yourself? If you're like me, you probably do it every day, convinced you can work, take care of your family, and save the world all before bedtime. With exercise, your unattainable goal may be to lose more weight than is healthy, schedule more exercise than you can handle, or change the basic structure of your body to look like a celebrity or movie star. The key is to work with the body you have under the circumstances you live in rather than an idealized version of your life and body.

Make goals realistic. Being realistic about what you want to accomplish is crucial for your success. If your goal is to exercise at 5:00 A.M. every day and you usually sleep until 7:00 A.M., is that realistic? You might do it once or twice, but after a few days of feeling cranky and tired, you might give up altogether. A more realistic goal might be to get up fifteen minutes earlier for a short workout and gradually add more time as you get used to it. Setting realistic goals is probably the most important part of the goal-setting process because it will require you to figure out what you'll really do rather than what you think you should do.

Make goals time oriented. In other words, if you have a weight-loss goal, you should also have a date to lose that weight. If you don't set a deadline for yourself, you may never get started—if you can start your workouts anytime, why start now? Just make sure the deadline you set is reasonable. For weight-loss goals, setting a time frame can be difficult since we only have so much control over how quickly we lose weight, but the next section will give you the basics of how weight loss works.

There are other things you can do to make reaching your goals a reality. In addition to setting SMART goals, try some of the following methods to ensure your success:

- **Write down your goals.** This helps you get clear on what you want to accomplish. Use the Goal Worksheet form on pages 39–40 or make your own form and keep it handy to motivate yourself.

WHAT'S HOT

▶ One growing fitness trend we've seen in the past few years is functional fitness—choosing workouts that help us function better in daily life. What a novel idea, right? Being more functional in your life is an excellent goal to have because it's motivating and measurable. Maybe you want to be able to pick up your kids without throwing out your back or go up the stairs without getting winded. What functional goals could you set for yourself?

- **Tell others about your goals.** You can get support and be held accountable for reaching your goals.
- **Track your progress.** Check in with yourself on a regular basis to see how you're doing and what you need to change.
- **Be flexible and realistic.** You won't always be able to stick with your scheduled workouts or eat healthy. Be aware that you may have setbacks.
- **Reward yourself.** Anytime you reach a goal, no matter how small, reward yourself for a job well done. It might be something small, like a new song for your MP3 player, or, for bigger goals, you could schedule a massage or a weekend trip. Celebrating every success feels good and reminds you that you're getting there.

The following is a goal worksheet that will help you keep track of your goals and plans for reaching them. There are spots for up to five goals, but you can write down fewer or more if you like. Make a copy of this sheet and keep it handy. Just reviewing your goals every once in a while will reaffirm your desire to reach them.

Date: _____

My health and fitness goals are:

1. _____
2. _____
3. _____
4. _____
5. _____

My deadlines for reaching these goals are:

1. _____
2. _____
3. _____
4. _____
5. _____

I will take the following steps to reach my goals:

1. _____
2. _____
3. _____
4. _____
5. _____

6. _____

7. _____

8. _____

9. _____

10. _____

I will use the following tools to track my progress:

_____

_____

_____

_____

_____

_____

My reward(s) for reaching my goals will be:

_____

_____

_____

_____

_____

_____

Losing Weight

You may have a number of things you want to accomplish as you get in shape, but losing weight often tops the list. With so many Americans sitting more than ever before and about 60 percent of us overweight, it isn't surprising that most people want to lose weight. The problem many beginners have is that their weight-loss goals aren't realistic. Most of us don't set goals that match our body, lifestyle, and fitness level but, instead, focus on an ideal body or an ideal workout schedule that's out of reach.

Another tendency is to have unrealistic expectations about how quickly we should be losing weight. I once worked with a client who, after seven weeks of exercise and watching her diet, lost 5 pounds. Instead of being excited about it, she showed up for her personal training session in tears, wondering why she hadn't lost more weight. When I pointed out that she was losing weight and that's exactly what we wanted, she shouted, "But it's only five pounds!" Her unrealistic expectations made her feel like a failure, even though she had proof she was on her way to reaching her goals. If weight loss is what you're after, understanding how it works can help you set the right goals and know what to expect so you don't get discouraged.

It's important to know how weight loss works. At its simplest, losing weight is about burning more calories than you eat. Obviously, if it were that simple, we'd all be thin and I'd be out of a job. But losing weight isn't as hard at it seems, it just takes some work and, most importantly, it takes patience. First, you should have a basic understanding of how weight loss works so you can set realistic goals in a reasonable time frame.

To lose 1 pound of fat, you would need to burn an extra 3,500 calories over and above your basal metabolic rate (BMR). Your BMR is the number of calories your body needs each day to function and is calculated by using height, weight, age, and gender. You can use the following formula to calculate your BMR:

For Women: BMR = 655 + (4.35 × weight in pounds) + (4.7 × height in inches) − (4.7 × age)
For Men: BMR = 66 + (6.23 × weight in pounds) + (12.7 × height in inches) − (6.8 × age)

For example, if you're a thirty-five-year-old male who is 6'0" tall and weighs 220 pounds, your BMR equation would look like this:

66 + (6.23 × 220 pounds) + (12.7 × 72 inches) − (6.8 × 35) = 2113

Most experts recommend losing about ½ to 2 pounds a week to ensure you're losing fat (losing more may cause you to lose muscle tissue as well). By following these guidelines, you would need to burn an extra 500 calories each day with both diet and exercise to lose one pound a week. To lose two pounds a week, you'd have to burn an extra 1,000 calories. That sounds reasonable, doesn't it? You could cut 250 food calories a day and burn off 250 with exercise, right? But where the problem comes in is that, first, you have to do that every single day (no cheat days allowed) to lose a pound in a week. Second, it isn't always easy to determine exactly how many calories you're burning with exercise.

Understanding that weight loss is sometimes two steps forward (you exercised and ate right for three days) and one step back (you had an extra piece of cake at the office party) can help you keep your expectations in check.

One of the simplest ways to approach weight loss is to reduce your calories by adjusting your diet and starting a daily exercise program. With this approach, you wouldn't be counting calories or

▶ The idea behind losing weight—eat less and move more—seems simple. If that's the case, why do we have so much trouble dropping extra pounds? My article "10 Reasons It's Hard to Lose Weight" discusses different factors that affect weight loss, such as your attitude about exercise, how you eat, and how you move each day. By understanding what might be holding you back, you can take charge of your weight loss and health. Check it out at http://about .com/exercise/weightloss.

keeping track of any numbers, but focusing more on being healthy and letting the weight loss happen in its own time. If you have a specific weight-loss goal and a specific time frame, you may need to follow a more complex plan to track your calories and your weight loss.

Here are some basic steps for getting started on your weight-loss strategy:

1. Calculate your BMR. If the equation given previously involves too much math and you'd like a simpler way to calculate your BMR, you can use an online calculator such as the one available at FitWatch.com (www.fitwatch.com/qkcalc/bmr.html). Be aware that the number you get is just an estimate and won't be exact. You may need to experiment over time to figure out how many calories you need to eat to fuel your body while still maintaining weight loss.

2. Determine how many calories you're burning with exercise or other activities. There are a number of formulas used to estimate calories burned for different activities, but you don't have to wade through complicated calculations. There are a number of online calculators to help you estimate how many calories you burn each day, such as my Calorie Calculator at http://about.com/exercise/caloriecalc.

3. Determine how many calories you burn through the thermic effect of food (TEF). Your body uses energy to help you digest your meals. To determine your TEF, you'll need to know how many calories you eat each day and multiply that number by 10 percent. For example, if you eat 2,000 calories a day, your TEF would be 200 calories.

4. Determine how many calories you're eating each day. This step is explained more thoroughly in Chapter 10, but in general, it starts with keeping a food journal and by measuring what you

I've lowered my calorie intake, but I'm not losing weight. What can I do?

▶ Reducing your calories is important for losing weight, but you don't want to go too low. Lowering your calories too far below your BMR or below about 1,000 can actually hurt your efforts to lose weight as your body goes into starvation mode. Food is fuel for your body, and eating regularly throughout the day can keep your metabolism going and your body functioning more efficiently.

eat and reading labels, adding up how many calories you're eating every day.

5. Add the numbers in steps 1, 2, and 3 and compare that sum to the number you calculated in step 4. If you're eating more than you're burning, you'll need to reduce your calories if you want to lose weight.

If you want to lose weight, set specific goals. When it comes to setting your weight-loss goals, one approach is to go by the numbers. Some options include:

- **Lower your body mass index (BMI).** If your BMI is over 25, you might set a goal for lowering that number to somewhere between 18.5 and 24.9. For example, if you're 5'8" and weigh 200 pounds, your BMI would be over 30 and your long-term goal might be to lose about 40 pounds.
- **Lose inches around the waist.** If your waist-hip ratio is higher than .8 for women or higher than 1.0 for men, losing inches may be your long-term goal. Similarly, if your abdominal girth is more than 35 inches for women and 40 inches for men, getting those measurements below the redline can be a goal.
- **Lose body fat.** If you're tracking your body-fat percentage, another approach would be to lower your body fat into a healthy range for your gender: 25–31 percent for women and 18–25 percent for men.
- **Improve your health.** If you have high blood pressure, high cholesterol, or are at risk for heart disease or diabetes, experts say that losing just 5–10 percent of your current weight can help you manage these issues. If you weigh 195 pounds, your goal would be to lose about 10–20 pounds.

These numbers cover the broad spectrum of weight loss and can be helpful in tracking your progress, but what about changing how your body looks? What about thinner thighs, flatter abs, and tighter buns? How much weight should you lose if you want to look good in a bathing suit? These goals fall under what I call the spot-training goals, and I hate to break it to you, but setting these kinds of goals may lead only to disappointment.

The Problem with Spot Training

"How do I get flat abs?" This is the single most frequent question I get, followed by how to get thin thighs, how to get rid of saddlebags, and how to reduce that annoying underarm flab. There's nothing wrong with wanting to lose fat from those stubborn areas of the body; we all want to look good, and we all have places where we store excess fat. The problem with these spot-training goals is that they go against the SMART principles. Unfortunately, spot training, or trying to change a specific body part with certain exercises, simply doesn't work.

Your body stores and loses fat in a certain order based on your genetic makeup and hormones, among other things. If your body is genetically predisposed to store excess fat around the belly, that may be one of the last places you end up losing the fat. Even if you do see improvements, you may not be able to lose all the fat there without taking your body fat to unhealthy or unsustainable levels. In other words, your body is in charge of how and when the fat comes off. That means ab exercises won't reduce the fat around your belly, nor will squats or leg lifts reduce the fat around your hips or thighs. Now your question might be, if those exercises don't work, then why am I doing them at all?

Those exercises do work and they are important for getting in shape. Strength-training exercises help you build lean muscle, which is essential for losing fat and shaping your body. But it's also essential for you to set realistic goals for yourself. If your body stores excess fat around your gut, having a goal to have abs like Tom Cruise or Madonna may be out of your genetic reach. Instead, set a goal to make your abs look the best they can within your body's parameters.

Take care when setting goals related to your appearance. There's nothing wrong with wanting to look better, and you'll certainly see improvements when you start exercising … but those improvements will be based on what your body is capable of.

Healthy Lifestyle Goals

Losing weight is a popular goal for many people, but believe it or not, there are other reasons to get in shape, and quality of life is probably the best reason there is. Exercising regularly can do all kinds of good things for you that can make your life better every day, like giving you more energy, making you more alert, helping you sleep better, and protecting you from illness and disease.

But exercise isn't the only way to improve your quality of life, and, in fact, having healthy lifestyle goals along with your weight-loss goals can be a great motivator for staying on track. Weight loss can be a slow process, but healthy lifestyle goals often offer immediate results. Plus, people who focus more on health and less on the scale often find long-term success at weight loss without all the obsessing and worry.

Being healthy can have a broad definition, but in general, it means you take care of yourself in every part of your life, from how much you sleep to how you manage stress. Below are some healthy lifestyle goals to consider adding to your list:

- Stop smoking
- Eat more fruits and veggies
- Cut out the trans fats

ELSEWHERE ON THE WEB

▶ If you're busy and stressed, you may have trouble going to sleep or staying asleep, and sleep deprivation can contribute to weight gain. To learn more about just how sleep deprived you are, take the Sleep Deprivation Screening Quiz at http://about.com/sleepdisorders/sleepquiz. Then browse around the site to get some helpful tips for getting more sleep. One great option is to take short power naps during the day to refresh and rejuvenate.

- Drink more water and less soda
- Sit less and move more
- Limit alcohol
- Get enough sleep
- Manage stress

Of all the goals above, the most important is to quit smoking. If you smoke, you already know the negative effects and that quitting can add healthy years to your life. Other important health goals that can have a direct effect on your weight loss include getting enough sleep and learning how to manage your stress in healthy ways.

Too often, people think that losing weight is about exercise and diet. While that's true to some degree, getting too little sleep and dealing with chronic stress can stall your weight loss, and it can even contribute to weight gain.

If you're sleep deprived, meaning you get less than eight hours of sleep on a regular basis, you tend to be less active. That's not surprising . . . who wants to exercise after getting only four or five hours of sleep? But that's not all. Some studies have shown that sleep deprivation can actually lower appetite-suppressing hormones so you feel hungrier and eat more.

Stress can also contribute to weight gain. In the last few years, experts have found a connection between abdominal fat and stress, noting that stress causes the release of the hormone cortisol, which can cause an increase in abdominal fat. Stress has also been linked to a number of other health problems, like diabetes, heart disease, and depression. Learning how to manage stress is critical if you want to be healthy and lose weight. Exercise is a great tool for reducing stress (you knew I was going to say that, didn't you?), but there are some other great tools as well, such as meditating, deep breathing, yoga, massage, and spending time each day relaxing.

Another part of being healthy is movement. Structured cardio and strength training are important, but a healthy lifestyle is also about what you do all day long, not just during exercise time. Experts have found that lean people don't necessarily have a high metabolism but are often slimmer simply because they move around more throughout the day. The great thing about this is that you can make subtle changes toward being more active without changing clothes, sweating, or going to a gym. Below are some simple ways you can add more movement into your life:

- Stand up while you work
- Sit on an exercise ball at work or while you watch TV
- Set an alarm to get up every hour and take a five-minute walk
- Pace while you talk on the phone
- Start a nightly tradition of walking with your family after dinner
- Avoid escalators, elevators, and moving walkways whenever possible

What ideas could you come up with to move more throughout your day? Make a list and see how many you can check off by the end of the day.

Start with Short-Term Goals

Setting a fitness goal is easy—the hard part is figuring out what you'll do to reach it. You can make it easier on yourself by mapping out the steps you'll take on a daily, weekly, and monthly basis. You may have a long-term goal to lose 50 pounds, but that's so far in the future, you may have trouble staying motivated on a daily basis. But if you break that down into smaller, simpler steps, you force yourself to focus on what you're doing right now rather than what will happen in the next six months or year. Think of it this way: You can't lose 50 pounds in the next week, but you could fit in three or four workouts and eat a healthy breakfast each day. Those workouts and dietary changes, followed consistently, are what will lead to your weight-loss goals.

Start by taking your long-term goal and breaking it down into monthly chunks. Think about what you want to accomplish in the next four weeks. For example, to lose 50 pounds, you know you need to exercise regularly and eat fewer calories each day. So, your monthly goal might be to establish a regular exercise routine three to five days a week and to start keeping a food journal and finding ways to reduce your calories each day.

With your monthly goal in mind, break it down even further into weekly goals. Using the example above, your goal for the week would be to plan and schedule your workouts (e.g., I'll walk for thirty minutes during my lunch hour on Monday, Wednesday, and Friday). To reduce your calories, your goal might be to buy a food journal or find a nutrition Web site where you can enter your foods each day and add up your calories.

If you really want to get into it, you can even break your weekly goals into daily goals—whatever works for you. Each week, you can check in with yourself to see if you reached all your goals. If you did not, try to come up with some ideas for what you could do differently to reach them the next week.

Getting Support for Your Goals

Now that you have some idea of how to set your fitness goals, you'll want to make sure you have a support system in place for following through with your plans. It's great to set a goal to exercise three times a week before work, but what if you have kids to take care of? What if your exercise time gets in the way of other obliga-

TOOLS YOU NEED

▶ Setting short-term goals can be confusing, but you can keep it simple by mapping out your plan for the week, day by day. For some ideas on how to set goals for yourself, check out my Sample Short-Term Weekly Goals Worksheet at http://about .com/exercise/shortterm goals. This sheet shows a weekly plan that includes cardio, strength training, and flexibility workouts, as well as sample nutrition goals for the week. Use this as a starting point to set your own weekly goals.

tions and duties? One way to handle these issues to get help from the people closest to you.

Get the family involved. Doing this on your own is hard, especially when you have work and family to take care of. Having support from your family can make the difference between reaching your goals and quitting before you ever get there. One approach would be to get the whole family on an exercise program, but if that isn't an option, at least sit down with them and talk about what you're trying to do and how they can help.

If it's difficult to schedule workouts around other family duties, could you have your spouse take care of the kids so you can fit in your workouts? Would your family be willing to go without the foods you find too tempting, like chips or sweets? Ask your family for help in coming up with ways to stay on track.

Gather support from friends and coworkers. It's easier to stick with your goals when you have people in your corner. Think about it: If you decide you want to eat healthier but you have to face that box of donuts your coworker brings to work each day, how hard will it be to stick with your goals?

As soon as you map out your goals, talk to the people close to you and tell them what you're doing. More importantly, ask them for their support in whatever way you need it.

If you need a watchdog or someone to call you on your behavior, you might ask a friend to call you or email you each day to ask if you did your workout. If you need help avoiding temptation like eating out too much or snacking on sweets, ask your coworkers to bring their lunch so you can all eat together, or have them hide the treats from you so you won't be tempted to eat them.

Get Linked

The following resources on my **About.com** *Exercise site will help you learn more about setting fitness goals that work with your specific needs, goals, and interests.*

HOW TO SET WEIGHT LOSS GOALS

Figuring out how much weight you need to lose and setting a reasonable time frame for losing it can be confusing. Taking the time to set reachable weight-loss goals is your first step toward success. This article provides tips for how to set goals that are attainable for your body and lifestyle.

 http://about.com/exercise/weightlossgoals

FITNESS MYTHS

Part of being successful at reaching fitness goals is knowing what you can expect from your exercise program. Exercise is a great tool for managing weight and getting fit, but it can't do everything. The more educated you are about what your body can do, the easier it will be to set and reach attainable goals. This article explains popular fitness myths that could be holding you back.

 http://about.com/exercise/fitnessmyths

IS THERE A SHORTCUT TO WEIGHT LOSS?

With all the weight-loss pills, gadgets, and infomercials, it's easy to believe that there's an easy way to lose weight. But the truth is, weight loss takes time, effort, discipline, and patience. This article describes the difference between shortcuts and genuine lifestyle changes to help you make the right choices for losing weight.

 http://about.com/exercise/shortcut

Chapter 4

Cardio Exercise

Cardio Basics

Whether your goal is to lose weight, build muscle, or improve your quality of life, cardio exercise is an essential part of a balanced exercise routine. Cardio exercise is any rhythmic movement that raises your heart rate over a period of time. By this definition, just about anything can count as cardio exercise if you can get your heart rate up and keep it up. Cardio exercise can help you:

- Burn calories and manage your weight
- Increase bone density
- Reduce your risk of heart disease, diabetes, and some types of cancer
- Lower cholesterol and blood pressure
- Manage symptoms of depression, anxiety, and stress
- Strengthen the heart and lungs
- Build confidence and improve self-esteem

About

- Have more energy throughout the day
- Sleep better

The nice thing about cardio is that you have a variety of activities to try, from things like walking and swimming to playing sports like basketball or tennis. Another great thing about cardio is that you have a number of elements you can manipulate to create a variety of workouts that keep you fit and stave off boredom. Those elements include the frequency, intensity, time, and type of cardio, or, here comes another acronym, FITT.

Workout Frequency and Duration

Now that you know how cardio exercise works, it's time to discuss how often you should do it and how long each individual workout should last. How often you do cardio exercise will depend on your goals, fitness level, and schedule. It goes without saying that doing some type of moderate cardio most days a week is a good idea whatever your goal is. One way to set your goals is to go by the exercise guidelines set out by the USDA:

- You should engage in regular physical activity for your physical and mental well-being, as well as to manage your weight.
- For health: Engage in thirty minutes of moderate-intensity exercise most days of the week.
- To lose weight or prevent weight gain: Do about sixty minutes of moderate- to vigorous-intensity exercise most days of the week while watching your calories.
- To sustain weight loss: Do sixty to ninety minutes of daily moderate-intensity exercise.

Before you freak out about trying to exercise for sixty to ninety minutes every day, it's important to realize that, first, how often you exercise each week will depend on how hard you work during your workouts, your schedule, your goals, and how much activity you do each day. If you're a beginner, you might want to start with three or four days a week and add on to that over time. One thing experts have found, however, is that beginners who do some type of activity every day of the week are more likely to stick to their exercise program.

Keep in mind that if you have a weight-loss goal but can't get the recommended exercise in, you may need to adjust your goal either by setting a different deadline or just focusing your attention on creating an exercise habit. Once you get that down, you can bring your weight-loss goal back into play.

And remember, you don't have to do your exercise all at once. If you have a busy schedule, you can split your workout into smaller chunks such as three 10-minute workouts or two separate 15-minute workouts. Heck, even five minutes of something is better than five minutes of nothing. Keep those guidelines in mind as you plan out your cardio strategy, but remember to keep your cardio goals SMART. Choose a frequency that's realistic for you, even if it doesn't exactly match those guidelines. You can always add more exercise as you get stronger, fitter, and more confident.

So, how long should each workout last? Take a look back at the USDA's exercise guidelines. It's important to remember that you don't have to start with ninety minutes of exercise, and in fact, you shouldn't start with that much exercise if you're a beginner. Your best bet is to start with the baseline recommendation, thirty minutes of moderate activity each day, and if that's too much for your body or your schedule, simply start with what you can do and remember you can always improve on that over time. Something is always better than nothing!

WHAT'S HOT

▶ Got ten minutes? If so, you can burn up to and over 100 calories with just ten minutes of exercise, if you work hard at it. Try running, jumping rope, or kickboxing drills, or find a nearby hill and walk or run up as fast as you can, recovering by walking back down. For more ideas on how you can burn more calories in less time, check out my article "Shake Up Your Workout and Burn 100 Calories in 10 Minutes," at http://about.com/exercise/burncalories.

Looking at all the elements we've covered—frequency, intensity, and type of activity—you'll start to understand that the duration of your workouts will often depend on these other factors. If you're walking every day at a moderate intensity, your workouts might last around thirty to sixty minutes. On the other hand, if you're doing high-intensity cardio workouts in the upper end of your target heart-rate zone, your workouts may last only about twenty or so minutes.

As mentioned in the section on intensity, it's best to have a variety of workouts. A typical setup might be one high-intensity workout; one long, slow workout; and then two or three medium-length, medium-intensity workouts. When you're just starting out with an exercise program, it's less important how fast you go; your first order of business is to build endurance in your heart and body, so focus more on sustaining the workout. When you can do that, then you can work on your pace and intensity.

Workout Intensity

The next element to consider is the intensity of your cardio workouts. The USDA's guidelines suggest moderate-intensity and vigorous-intensity activities, but what exactly does that mean? The American College of Sports Medicine (ACSM) has broken down the different levels of intensity into three categories, all based on a percentage of your maximum heart rate (MHR):

- Moderate activity is between 55 and 69 percent of MHR
- Vigorous or hard activity is between 70 and 89 percent of MHR
- Very hard activity is 90 percent or more of MHR

To determine your maximum heart rate, you can subtract your age from 220. Then take that number and multiply it by the

ELSEWHERE ON THE WEB

▶ Working out on gym machines can get a little boring, even if the machine you're using offers programs. If you've got an MP3 or CD player, consider guided cardio workouts like those offered by Cardio Coach (www.cardiocoach.com). Cardio Coach offers more than six guided workouts you can download to your MP3 player. The interval workouts can be done on any machine (or outside) and your cardio coach provides motivation and encouragement to keep you going.

percentage of MHR to figure out what heart rate corresponds to different intensity levels. For example, if you're forty-seven years old, your calculation would look like this:

220 – 47 = 173 MHR
173 × .55 = 95 beats per minute, the low end of your moderate activity zone
173 × .69 = 119 beats per minute, the high end of your moderate activity zone

This formula gives you a rough estimate of maximum heart rate, but it won't be entirely accurate, so use these numbers as a guideline only.

Another formula that offers a bit more detail is the Karvonen formula, which determines heart rate based on your heart rate reserve (HRR) and a training range that is between 50 percent and 85 percent of your HRR. This all sounds very complicated, but the formula is fairly simple, although you will need to find your resting heart rate (RHR) to use this formula. To find your RHR, take your pulse for one full minute either before you get out of bed in the morning or after resting quietly for at least thirty minutes:

220 – age = maximum heart rate (MHR)
MHR – resting heart rate (RHR) = heart rate reserve (HRR)
HRR × 50% or 85% = your training zone %
training zone % + RHR = target heart rate zone

Here's an example for a thirty-year-old person with a resting heart rate of 60 beats per minute:

220 – 30 = 190
190 – 60 (RHR) = 130

ELSEWHERE ON THE WEB

▶ There's been some speculation in the past few years that the MHR formula, 220 minus age, isn't very accurate because the number, 220, is based on a sedentary person. If you're fit, using that formula may not work for you, and even the Karvonen formula may be a little off. Steven's Creek offers a formula that takes into account different MHRs for different fitness levels: http://stevens creek.com/goodies/hr.shtml.

130 × 50% (low end) or 85% (high end) = 65 – 110
65 + 60 (RHR) = 125 beats per minute
110 + 60 (RHR) = 170 beats per minute
Target heart rate zone = 125 to 170 beats per minute.

Gee, you didn't realize there'd be so much math, did you? The good news is that there are online calculators for finding your target heart rate zone, but it's always a good idea to have a little knowledge about what's behind these formulas and what they mean.

Now that you have a target heart rate zone, how do you actually monitor your heart rate? One option is by using a heart rate monitor. A heart rate monitor is simply a watch that comes with a strap you wrap around your chest during exercise. This strap sends a signal to your watch, allowing you to see a continuous reading of your heart rate. There are a variety of monitors out there for every budget and every type of exerciser, from basic models that just measure heart rate, to high-tech models that measure everything from heart rate and calories to pace, speed, and time spent in your zone. You can find heart rate monitors at most sporting-goods stores and discount stores.

If you don't want to bother with formulas or heart rate monitors, there are other, simpler, ways to monitor the intensity of your workouts. The simplest method is the talk test. With this test, you only have to ask yourself one question: Am I able to carry on a conversation? If you can talk during your workout without becoming breathless, you're most likely working at a moderate intensity.

Another method to monitor intensity is using a perceived exertion scale to measure your rate of perceived exertion (RPE). Perceived exertion is simply how hard you feel you're working during exercise. It's a subjective measure and will differ from person to person, but studies have found that it's an accurate way to monitor your exercise intensity. The standard scale most people use

ELSEWHERE ON THE WEB

▶ There are so many heart rate monitors to choose from, you may feel overwhelmed. Before you buy one, consider your needs. If you just want to track your heart rate, choose a basic model. If you're a serious athlete who wants to track workouts, you might get a model that allows you to download information to your computer. Above all, do some research. You can find reviews of heart rate monitors at Consumer Search (www.consumersearch.com).

is the Borg Scale, which ranges from 6 to 20, 6 being the easiest and 20 being the hardest. Using this scale, 6 would be the equivalent of doing nothing, and 20 would be working at your absolute maximum. A moderately intense activity would fall somewhere between 12 and 13.

A simplified perceived exertion scale can range from 1 to 10:

- **Level 1:** I'm watching TV and eating bonbons.
- **Level 2:** I'm comfortable and could maintain this pace all day long.
- **Level 3:** I'm still comfortable but am breathing a bit harder.
- **Level 4:** I'm sweating a little but feel good and can carry on a conversation effortlessly.
- **Level 5:** I'm just above comfortable, am sweating more, and can still talk easily.
- **Level 6:** I can still talk but am slightly breathless.
- **Level 7:** I can still talk, but I don't really want to. I'm sweating like a pig.
- **Level 8:** I can grunt in response to your questions and can only keep this pace for a short time period.
- **Level 9:** I am probably going to die.
- **Level 10:** I am dead.

Using this scale, a moderate pace would be around 4 or 5, while a vigorous pace would fall between 7 and 9.

When it comes to losing weight, you may have heard that you should stay within your fat-burning zone to get the most out of your workouts. The fat-burning zone, which would roughly match a moderate-intensity workout, is actually somewhat of a myth. Working at lower intensities for longer periods of time can help you burn a larger percentage of fat. But working at a higher intensity will help you burn overall calories, which is what you want if

ASK YOUR GUIDE

What's the best way to monitor my exercise intensity?

▶ My favorite method is a combination of heart rate and perceived exertion. While wearing a heart rate monitor, determine how hard you're working at different intensities by using perceived exertion. At the same time, make a note of your heart rate. By matching heart rate to perceived exertion, you can tweak your target heart rate zone to make workouts more efficient. For more information, check out my article "Find Your Target Heart Rate," at http://about .com/exercise/targetheart rate.

you're trying to lose weight. That isn't to say that going slower is bad or that you should kill yourself during every cardio workout. What it means is that you should have a mix of workouts at various intensities so you can challenge your heart, energy systems, and body in different ways.

One way to incorporate high-intensity exercise into your workouts is to do interval training. In this type of workout, you alternate between periods or distances of high-intensity exercise and low-intensity exercise to recover. An example of this would be to walk for two minutes and run or sprint for thirty seconds, alternating between the two several times. This is also a great way to ease into a running program if you're a beginner. You'll find a variety of interval and walk/run workouts at the end of this chapter to give you an idea of how it works.

Types of Cardio

When it comes to cardio exercise, there's no limit to your choices. If you're a beginner, walking is almost always a good choice since you don't need any fancy equipment (other than a good pair of shoes), there's no learning curve, and you can do it anywhere without a lot of fuss. But because walking is such a familiar activity, your body is very good at it, so you may have to work a bit harder to get your heart rate up if walking is your exercise of choice. Some options include:

- Adding short spurts of jogging or running to your walk, which can help you burn more calories
- Adding hills or inclines throughout your workouts
- Using walking poles to work the upper body and burn more calories
- Every so often, speeding up and walking as fast as you can

▶ Vacations aren't just an excuse to laze around on the beach anymore. These days, more and more people are taking walking vacations so they can see all the sights while avoiding vacation weight gain. Walking is the perfect way to get to know the area while staying active. Looking for ideas on how to plan a walking vacation? Wendy Bumgardner, About.com's Walking Guide, tells you how in her article "Take a Walking Vacation": http://about.com/walking/walking vacation.

One thing you want to avoid is carrying weights in your hands or strapped to your ankles as you walk. Many people do this to burn more calories, but you actually put yourself at risk for an injury. If adding weight is something you're determined to do, it's best to wear a weighted vest so that the extra weight is more evenly distributed throughout the body and your joints aren't at risk. Another no-no is holding onto the rails while you're walking on the treadmill. If you've never been on one before, you may need the rails at first, but you shouldn't take your speed and/or incline so high that you're holding on for dear life. Not only does that cheat you out of burning calories, it also interferes with your body's natural biomechanics and can strain your upper body.

Running is another good choice if you want an accessible exercise that can really help you zip through the calories. If you're a walker or you've never tried running before, it's best to ease into a running routine by alternating periods of walking and running. The simplest way to do this is to head out the door and start with a brisk walk for about five minutes. When you're warm, move into a slow jog until you get breathless or need a break. Walk until you've recovered and then run again, alternating for about twenty or so minutes. Each week, increase your running time and decrease your walking time until you can run continuously for the desired length of time.

Running and walking are just two options for you to choose from. Other popular cardio activities might include cycling; swimming; kickboxing; step or hi/lo aerobics; hiking; rowing; or playing sports like basketball, handball, or soccer. It's great to do a variety of exercises once you get into a consistent routine to avoid getting bored or getting a repetitive strain injury from doing the same type of movement over and over.

ELSEWHERE ON THE WEB

▶ To start a running program, its easier if you walk before you run. Taking the time to condition your body will make the experience more pleasurable and help you avoid common ailments like shin splints and side stitches. Jeff Galloway, one of the most well-known and decorated runners of our time, describes simple steps for easing into running as well as moving into different stages of running on his Web site. Check out the section for Beginner runners at www .jeffgalloway.com/training/ beginners.html.

Don't forget, cardio exercise is anything that gets your heart rate up and that you can maintain for periods of time, so you aren't just limited to cardio machines or fitness classes. For example, shoveling snow, cutting the grass (with a push mower, of course), running up and down the stairs, and dancing wildly around the house to your favorite music are just a few activities that can get your heart rate up if you work hard enough.

The most important thing is to choose activities you enjoy, and the only way to do that is to be willing to try different things. Keep in mind that anytime you try a new activity, it will feel challenging and strange. Give it some time before you decide you don't like something.

Cardio Workouts

As mentioned, a great way to burn calories and increase endurance is to try interval training, where you alternate high- and low-intensity intervals throughout your workout. The following are a variety of cardio workouts, from beginning intervals to a walk/run workout, to give you an idea of how interval training can work and how to get started. These workouts range from beginner level to intermediate and can be done outside or using any type of cardio machine. The high-intensity intervals include increasing your pace, your resistance/incline, or both, and the intensity level is based on the perceived exertion scale detailed above on a scale from 1 to 10. During most workouts, your RPE will range from 4 to 8.

Beginner Interval Workout

This 20-minute Beginner Interval Workout involves high- and low-intensity intervals that can be done on any cardio machine or outside. Simply increase your speed during the intensity intervals until you're slightly breathless and working at an RPE of about 7 or 8. Lower your pace during the low-intensity segments until you feel fully recovered for the next intensity interval.

BEGINNER INTERVAL WORKOUT

Time	Activity	Intensity Level
3 minutes	Move at an easy pace to warm up	3–4
2 minutes	Speed up to a brisk pace	4
3 minutes	Increase your pace to reach your baseline speed	5
30 seconds	Increase your pace so you're working hard	7–8
3 minutes	Decrease your pace back to baseline	5
30 seconds	Increase your pace so you're working hard	7–8
3 minutes	Decrease your pace back to baseline	5
5 minutes	Decrease to an easy pace for a cooldown	3–4

Walk/Run Workout for Beginners

The following 25-minute workout is a beginner running program that alternates walking and running on a treadmill or outside. The speeds listed are just suggestions, so adjust your speed until you're working at the appropriate perceived exertion or adjust the intervals to walk longer or run longer to fit your fitness level.

WALK/RUN WORKOUT FOR BEGINNERS

Time	Activity	Intensity Level
5 minutes	Warm up: 2.5–3.0 mph	4
3 minutes	Brisk walk: 3.0–3.5 mph	5
1 minute	Easy jog: 4.0–4.5 mph	7
3 minutes	Brisk walk: 3.0–3.5 mph	5
1 minute	Jog: 4.2–4.5 mph	8
3 minutes	Brisk walk: 3.0–3.5 mph	5
30 seconds	Jog: 4.2–4.7 mph	8
3 minutes	Brisk walk: 3.0–3.5 mph	5
30 seconds	Jog: 4.2–4.7 mph	8
2 minutes	Brisk walk: 3.0–3.5 mph	5
3 minutes	Cool down at an easy pace	3–4

Speed/Resistance Interval Training

The following 30-minute interval workout is a bit more advanced, involving both speed and resistance/incline intervals and ranging from 5 to 9 RPE. It can be done on any cardio machine or you can do it outside by using nearby hills or just staying with speed intervals.

SPEED/RESISTANCE INTERVAL TRAINING

Time	Activity	Intensity Level
5 minutes	Warm up at an easy pace	4
2 minutes	Increase pace to your baseline	5
1 minute	Increase resistance/incline until you're working somewhat hard	6–7
1 minute	Lower resistance and increase speed to work hard	8
2 minutes	Go back to baseline to recover	5
1 minute	Increase resistance/incline	6–7
1 minute	Decrease resistance and increase speed	8
2 minutes	Go back to baseline	5
1 minute	Increase resistance/incline	7
1 minute	Decrease resistance and increase speed	9
2 minutes	Go back to baseline	5
1 minute	Increase resistance/incline	7
1 minute	Decrease resistance and increase speed	9
2 minutes	Go back to baseline	5
1 minute	Increase resistance/incline	7
1 minute	Decrease resistance and increase speed	8
5 minutes	Cool down at an easy pace	5

Intermediate Interval Training

This workout is more than 30 minutes long and involves both speed and resistance/incline intervals that can be done on any machine or outside. During the intensity intervals, you'll be increasing your speed or resistance every 20 seconds for a total of 2 minutes. By the end of the interval, you should be working at an RPE of about 7 to 9, so adjust speed/incline as needed.

INTERMEDIATE INTERVAL TRAINING

Time	Activity	Intensity Level
5 minutes	Warm up	4–5
2 minutes	Baseline pace	5
2 minutes	Increase resistance/incline 1% / 30 seconds	7–8
2 minutes	Decrease resistance/incline 1% / 30 seconds	6–7
1 minute	Baseline pace	5
2 minutes	Increase speed .5 mph / 30 seconds	7–8
2 minutes	Decrease speed .5 mph / 30 seconds	6–7
1 minute	Baseline pace	5
2 minutes	Increase resistance/incline 1% / 30 seconds	7–8
2 minutes	Decrease resistance/incline 1% / 30 seconds	6–7
1 minute	Baseline pace	5
2 minutes	Increase speed .5 mph / 30 seconds	7–8
2 minutes	Decrease speed .5 mph / 30 seconds	6–7
1 minute	Baseline pace	5
30 seconds	Sprint as fast as you can	9
1 minute	Baseline pace	5
30 seconds	Sprint as fast as you can	9
5 minutes	Cool down at an easy pace	3–4

Get Linked

The following resources on my **About.com** *Exercise site will give you a greater understanding of how to set up a cardio program based on your fitness level, goals, and interests.*

CARDIO 101

Understanding the basic elements of cardio exercise can help you set up a cardio program to fit your schedule, fitness level, and goals. This article offers details about each part of a cardio program to help you choose activities you enjoy and make sure you're getting the most out of your exercise time.

 http://about.com/exercise/cardio101

HOW TO MONITOR YOUR EXERCISE INTENSITY

Staying within your cardio training zone is essential for burning calories, losing weight, and conditioning your heart. This article will teach you more about how you can monitor your exercise intensity so you can set up the most efficient and effective workouts for your goals and schedule.

 http://about.com/exercise/intensity

CARDIO WORKOUTS

Variety is one of the most important elements of a good cardio program. By training your body with new activities and at different levels of intensity, you'll keep your body challenged and your mind interested. This index lists a variety of free cardio workouts for every level of fitness.

 http://about.com/exercise/cardioworkouts

Chapter 5

Strength Training

Strength-Training Basics

If your goal is to lose weight, get in shape, or just be healthier, you know that cardio exercise is an important tool for doing that. But did you know that strength training is just as important as cardio for weight loss? Or that strength training can save you from that drop in metabolism that happens as you age? There are still plenty of people who think strength training is just for bodybuilders, but incorporating weights into your weekly routine can:

- Build lean muscle, which is more metabolically active than fat
- Reduce body fat, for a healthier body composition
- Increase bone density
- Increase muscular strength and endurance
- Help protect you from injuries
- Improve strength and power for sports
- Build confidence and self-esteem
- Improve balance, coordination, and stability

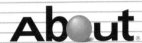

How can I build bigger muscles and lose fat at the same time?

▶ Building big muscles and losing fat are two different and conflicting goals. To gain muscle weight, you need to eat more calories than you burn. To lose fat, you need to burn more calories than you eat. You can still get stronger while losing weight, but by reducing your food intake, you won't be taking in the calories your muscles need to grow bigger.

Most people know how to do cardio exercise, but strength training can be confusing. There are so many exercises and machines, so many choices for how many sets, reps, and weights—where do you start? Setting up a program is a step-by-step process that starts with knowing the basic principles of strength training. These principles are designed to help you set up a program that is efficient, effective, and safe for reaching your goals.

1. **Overload.** The purpose of lifting weights is to get stronger and build lean muscle. The only way that can happen is if you overload your muscles—or challenge them with more weight than they can handle. When you do that, your muscles will grow stronger in order to handle that weight. To apply this principle to workouts, you want to make sure that you choose a weight that you can lift for *only* the desired number of reps. That means, if you're doing twelve biceps curls, you want to choose a weight you can lift only twelve times.

2. **Progression.** This principle is based on the fact that your body will adapt to the exercises you're doing—so you constantly have to progress and challenge your body if you want it to continue to get stronger and fitter. With weight training, that may mean changing weight, reps, sets, or your program as your body adapts to what you're doing. Typically, you want to change your strength program every four to six weeks to avoid strength and weight-loss plateaus.

3. **Specificity.** This principle simply means that you should train your body for what you want to achieve. If you want to be a bodybuilder, you should follow a program of heavy weights with fewer repetitions. If your goal is to lose fat, you wouldn't want to train like a bodybuilder, but have a more moderate approach to weight training, with plenty of cardio as well. If you're running a marathon, you'll need a strength-training

program that keeps you strong and fit for running but doesn't interfere with your training.

4. **Rest.** Your workouts are important in reaching your goals, but equally important is getting your rest. Your muscles need rest and recovery to grow, and in fact, it's during your rest days that your muscles rebuild themselves to become stronger. This means you don't want to work the same muscle groups two days in a row, and if you're lifting heavy, you may need more than one rest day between workouts.

Along with the principles behind strength training, you should also know what strength training can and can't do for your body. There are a number of weight-training myths floating around that may keep you from lifting weights or give you unrealistic expectations about what you can expect from lifting weights:

- **Myth:** Lifting weights will make you big and bulky. It's very difficult to build big muscles—ask any bodybuilder. If you're a woman, it's unlikely you'll gain large amounts of muscle since women usually don't have the levels of testosterone needed to do so. Even lifting heavy weights doesn't mean you'll put on pounds and pounds of muscle, so don't be afraid to go heavy and really challenge your body.
- **Myth:** Lifting weights will give you flat abs or thin thighs. Strength training isn't magic. You can't use strength-training moves to lose fat over certain areas of the body. But you can strengthen your body and build more lean muscle tissue, which will help raise your metabolism and improve your body composition.
- **Myth:** If you stop lifting weights, your muscle will turn to fat. Muscle and fat are two different types of tissue, and one can't become the other. If you stop lifting weights, muscle

doesn't disappear, but it can lose firmness, which may make you look and feel flabbier. Strength training is something you have to do consistently in order to get the most out of it.

- **Myth:** Strength training will reshape your muscles. You can't change the basic structure of your muscles with anything other than surgery. Muscles can get bigger or smaller, but strength training can't lengthen them or shorten them past where they attach to your bones.
- **Myth:** You should be sore after every workout. Being sore is normal if you're trying something new, but soreness is not necessarily an indicator of a good workout. If you're sore all the time, it may mean you're actually doing too much and should back off and take more rest days. To make sure you have a good workout, don't rely on soreness but on the intensity of the exercises while you're working out. If you follow the principles of strength training and make sure you're really lifting enough weight to become fatigued at the end of each set, you're on the right track.

Choosing Exercises

I've never counted them, but I would guess there are hundreds of strength-training exercises to choose from when setting up a strength-training program. That makes it difficult to figure out what exercises you should be doing. Are some better than others? How do you choose? The ACSM suggests in their strength-training guidelines that beginners choose a total of eight to ten exercises for the major muscle groups. That may seem vague, but as you learn more in the next few chapters about the muscle groups you should work and which exercises work those muscles, you'll find it's easy to set up a basic workout.

ELSEWHERE ON THE WEB

▶ You don't need a degree in anatomy and physiology to start a strength-training program, but knowing the muscles you're working, where they are, and how they work can give you a better understanding of which exercises to do and how to do them. ExRx (www.exrx.net/Exercise.html) is an excellent resource, providing detailed information about all the muscles of the body along with a database of exercises targeting those muscles.

The following is a list of standard exercises targeting the major muscle groups of the body:

- **Chest:** push-ups, chest press, chest fly
- **Upper and mid-back:** lat pull-downs, bent-over rows, seated row
- **Shoulders:** overhead press, lateral raise, front raise
- **Biceps:** biceps curls, hammer curls, concentration curls
- **Triceps:** kickbacks, triceps extensions, dips
- **Lower body:** squats, lunges, leg press, calf raises
- **Abs and lower back:** crunches, plank, back extensions

This list doesn't cover all the exercises you can do, but with the examples above and the guidelines to do eight to ten exercises, a beginner program might include the following exercises:

- Chest presses
- Lat pull-downs
- Overhead presses
- Biceps curls
- Kickbacks
- Leg presses
- Lunges
- Calf raises
- Crunches and back extensions

This basic program covers every part of your body and would be a good start for beginning exercisers.

Another general rule of thumb for choosing exercises is to do as many **compound movements** as possible. Compound movements are exercises that work more than one muscle group at a

Will cycling or using the stair-stepper make my butt bigger?

▶ Though bikes and stair-steppers offer resistance, it isn't enough to build big muscles in the glutes. To build muscles you have to overload them with more weight than they can handle, and cardio machines typically don't offer that level of resistance. In addition, during cardio exercise, your body relies on your endurance muscles slow-twitch muscle fibers rather than muscle fibers designed to grow larger fast-twitch muscle fibers.

time and involve more than one joint movement. These moves are great because they can save you time (the more muscles you involve, the more calories you can burn and the more weight you can lift), and they are often more functional since our bodies work as a whole and no one body part or muscle group is isolated during natural movement. Examples of compound movements would include squats, lunges, or barbell rows, just to name a few. Compound moves usually involve large and small muscle groups at the same time, so if you're short on time, you can skip exercises that work the small muscles (like the arms or calves) by making sure you're working them with compound moves. For example, lunges and squats will work the major muscles of the glutes and thighs along with the calves. A barbell row works the muscles of the back as well as the biceps.

Another aspect to consider is the sequence of your exercises. You'll find that most workouts follow a general pattern starting with larger muscles, like chest and back, and moving down to the smaller muscle groups, like shoulders and arms. The reason is that the most demanding exercises target the larger muscle groups, and you'll need the smaller muscles to help you get the most out of those exercises. If the smaller muscles are too tired, you may not be able to lift as much weight. But don't feel like you always have to do exercises in a certain order. Changing the sequence of exercises is often a great way to shake up your program, so try experimenting to see what feels right to you.

Choosing Resistance

Just like choosing your exercises, you also have a variety of options when choosing what type of resistance you use. The most popular are weight machines and free weights (dumbbells or barbells, for example), but what about cables or resistance bands? Which one is the best resistance to use? First, resistance training means you're lifting against some type of resistance; whether it comes from a dumbbell, a machine, or your two-year-old makes no difference to your muscles. The type of resistance you choose will be based on what you have available and what you're comfortable with.

There has long been a debate regarding machines and free weights: Is one better than the other? Both are effective for helping you reach your goals, and there's no reason you can't use both throughout your workouts since they each offer something different. But you'll find that most fitness experts, myself included, prefer free weights over machines in most situations because they allow you to work your body the way it works in day-to-day life.

However, machines can be great tools, especially for beginners. Most machines offer controlled movement and have a set pattern of motion, so if you're not sure how to do an exercise, the machine helps you stay on the right track and do the moves correctly. Machines can also provide support for your body so you can focus on getting your form down without involving the rest of your body. But that can also be a downside. By having all that support, you leave out other muscle groups that could help you stabilize your own body, thus helping you burn more calories while working your body in a more functional way. For example, a chest-press machine provides a padded backrest to support your back as you push the weight out. By switching to dumbbells, you suddenly have a weight in each hand and now have to use the muscles of your shoulders and arms to stabilize you as you push the weight up and down.

When you use free weights, you're using natural motion rather than the controlled motion offered by machines. For this reason, you'll often be using more muscle groups through a more natural range of motion when you use free weights. Another bonus of free weights is that they offer more options than a machine does. On a chest-press machine, there's only one thing you can do—sit

WHAT'S HOT

▶ Balance training has become part of the fitness culture as we focus more on exercises that enhance daily life. Having good balance is something we often take for granted, but as we get older, balance can be compromised if we aren't active. Many strength-training exercises help with balance, but you can also incorporate a little balance training into the things you do on a regular basis. For ideas, check out my article "How's Your Balance?" at http://about.com/exercise/balance.

ELSEWHERE ON THE WEB

▶ Figuring out how to use strength-training equipment can be difficult, but you can often find descriptions and pictures of exercises online to give you ideas of what you can do. Sissel, a company that makes a variety of exercise equipment, offers free pictures and descriptions of exercises you can try with exercise balls, resistance bands, inflatable disks, and other balance equipment. Visit www.sissel-online.com/exercisesmain.php.

on it and push the weight out and in. With dumbbells, you can do more variations, such as a flat chest press, an incline press, one arm at a time, or even chest presses with your knees up and feet off the floor. Free-weight exercises can often save time as well. With machines, you have to move from one machine to another to target different muscle groups; with free weights, you can often stay in the same area and even use the same weights for a variety of exercises. If you're a beginner, you might start with basic machine exercises and slowly incorporate more free-weight exercises as you get stronger and more comfortable with weight training.

But your choices don't just end with machines or dumbbells. Other options for resistance include resistance tubes or bands, cables, and even just your own body weight. Bands and cables offer a different kind of resistance that often feels harder. Gravity is involved with free weights, so you often get more resistance during one part of an exercise (pushing the weight up in a chest press) than the other (lowering the weight in a chest press). When you use bands or cables, there's constant tension during each part of the movement, which fires the muscle fibers in different ways and often makes exercises feel more difficult, providing you keep the tension high. This type of resistance also requires quite a bit of stabilization throughout the body, so you can work on balance, stability, and coordination at the same time you're building strength. With resistance bands or tubes, you also have control over the amount of tension throughout the exercise. This allows you to increase or decrease the resistance as needed.

Body-weight exercises can be a good choice for beginners or for when you're traveling. Exercises like push-ups, dips, squats, and lunges can help you work your body without much added equipment. Just remember the principle of overload: If you want your body to get stronger and fitter, you have to challenge it with more weight than it can handle. When the body-weight exercises get too easy, you'll need to add some type of resistance to increase the challenge.

Choosing Reps, Sets, and Weights

Once you've chosen your exercises and type of resistance, it's time to choose your repetitions (or reps), sets, and weights. Like the other elements of fitness, how many reps and sets you do will be based on your goals and your fitness level. The ACSM recommends that beginners stick with one set of eight to twelve reps to fatigue (meaning, you use enough weight that you can complete only the desired number of reps with good form), but there are different ranges of repetitions that focus on strength, muscle growth, and endurance.

In general, you get the most strength gains when you lift heavy weights between six and eight repetitions. For strength and hypertrophy, or bigger muscles, you should stay between eight and twelve repetitions. Lifting between twelve and sixteen repetitions will increase muscular endurance. But you're not limited to only one choice when it comes to choosing reps. Many exercisers focus on building strength and muscle for a period of time (8 to 12 reps) and then change their focus to endurance (12 to 16 reps) to keep their bodies challenged in different ways.

There is a rumor running around out there that using lighter weights for higher reps will tone the body and help you burn more fat. But there is a point of diminishing returns when you do too many reps with lighter weight. Science has found that, just like the heart has a training range most efficient for burning calories and building endurance, our muscles have a rep range where we can get the most strength and muscle gains (6 to 16 reps). When it comes to weight training, more reps aren't always better.

TOOLS YOU NEED

▶ If you travel, it can be tough to stay on track with exercise since you often don't have access to your usual equipment or schedule. It is possible to do challenging workouts in a hotel room with no equipment if you try some of the more intense body-weight exercises available or if you use what you have around, like your computer bag, for weight. For some ideas, try my No Equipment Travel Workout at http://about.com/exercise/travelworkout.

ELSEWHERE ON THE WEB

▶ Elite athletes often use a training method called periodization to divide their training programs so they focus on different areas of fitness, such as strength, endurance, speed, and rest as they get ready for competition. Periodization can be complicated, but regular exercisers can use the concept to create new workout programs every few weeks to keep the body challenged in new ways. You can learn more about periodization in Mistress Krista's article "Periodization," at www .stumptuous.com/cms/display article.php?aid=66.

The next question is, how many sets should you be doing? Read up on the subject and you'll find a variety of different opinions. As mentioned before, the ACSM recommends that beginners start with one set. But it suggests that multiset training (up to 3 sets) may offer more benefits as you become stronger and fitter, so once you've gotten started with a basic program of one-set training, you'll eventually want to add at least one more set to continue challenging your muscles in new ways. With my own workouts, I often follow a basic rule: The larger the muscle, the more sets I do. So, I may do three sets of exercises for the chest, back, and legs while just sticking with two sets of exercises for the shoulders, arms, and calves. Since many of the moves for the chest, back, and legs are compound and involve the smaller muscle groups, I don't need to work them quite as hard.

And don't forget the rest between sets, which is always important. In general, rest periods are usually between thirty seconds and two minutes, depending on the intensity of your workouts. For very heavy lifting, you'll want up to two minutes of rest between sets. For more moderate training, your rest may be between thirty and sixty seconds. If you're lifting light or doing body-weight exercises, you may need only a few seconds of rest between sets.

Finally, figure out how much weight you need for each exercise. There are some formal tests you can use based on a percentage of your one rep maximum (1 RM) for each exercise, but if you like things simple like I do, you can use the very scientific method of guessing. Here's a step-by-step approach you can use to determine how much weight you need for your exercises.

1. Pick up a light-medium weight and perform a warm-up set (about 16 reps) of the exercise.

2. If the weight felt light during the warm-up set, add about 3 to 5 pounds (or more if it felt very light) and perform another set, this time for your desired number of reps.

3. If you can continue lifting even after you reach the end of the set, increase the weight again for the next set or, if you're doing only two sets, make a note to increase the weight for your next workout.

4. Do the same for each exercise, making sure the weight you choose is enough that you can complete only the desired number of reps. You should be able to complete the set with good form, but the last rep should feel very difficult.

For example, say you're doing an overhead press and you started with 5 pounds. After the warm-up set, you move up to 8 pounds and do twelve repetitions. As you reach the last rep, you realize you could keep going, which means that weight was too light. For your next set, you might increase the weight to 10 or 12 pounds to add more intensity.

It may take some time and experimentation to find the right amount of weight to use, and you'll notice that some days you're stronger than others. Keeping a strength-training log is a great way to keep track of the weights you're using from week to week to decide when it's time to go heavier.

Setting Up a Strength Program

Now that you have all the elements of a basic strength-training program, you might be wondering how to put them together into something that makes sense. For beginners, ACSM recommends a total-body routine about two to three nonconsecutive days a week. More advanced exercisers may split their routines so that they're lifting for different muscle groups 4 or 5 days a week. It can be confusing figuring out how to schedule your strength-training workouts, but as long as you're following the strength-

ASK YOUR GUIDE

Why am I gaining weight after starting a strength-training program?

▸ If you're sure you're not eating too many calories, it's possible that you're gaining muscle faster than you're losing fat. This can result in an initial weight gain, but don't panic and don't stop lifting weights. That weight gain should correct itself over time if you continue to exercise and follow a healthy diet. Just make sure you're getting enough cardio exercise to encourage weight loss.

training principles (challenging all your muscle groups and allowing them to rest between workouts), there aren't any limits to what you can do. The following are just a few examples of typical strength-training routines to choose from:

- **Total Body.**
- **Upper Body and Lower Body.** Split your routine so that you're alternating upper-body exercises one day and lower-body exercises the next.
- **Push/Pull Split.** Another option is to do all push-type exercises one day (for example, squats, calf raises, bench press, overhead press, and dips) and pull-type exercises the next (like hamstring curls, lat pulldowns, upright rows, and biceps curls).
- **Three-Day Upper- and Lower-Body Split.** A typical version of this is day one: chest, shoulders, and triceps; day two: legs and abs; day three: back and biceps.

You can even lift weights for a different muscle group every day, if that's what works for you. All that matters is that you try to work each muscle group at least twice a week and give each muscle group at least forty-eight hours of rest before you work it again.

Whichever program you choose, you want to make sure you're following a few basic rules:

- **Warm up before workouts.** Your warm-up can be a few minutes of cardio or warm-up sets for each exercise you're doing.
- **Use good form.** Good form changes depending on what exercise you're doing, but for the most part, it means standing up straight; keeping your abs contracted; and lifting with slow, controlled movements.

TOOLS YOU NEED

▶ One mistake beginners often make is going too light in their strength-training workouts. There's nothing wrong with taking it easy during your first few workouts and allowing yourself time to learn the exercises and ease your body into training. But you should eventually work your way up so that you're lifting heavy enough to really challenge your muscles. For details, check out my article "Are You Lifting Enough Weight?" at http://about.com/exercise/liftingweight.

- **Don't use momentum.** If you find you have to swing your weights to lift them, you should lower the amount of weight you are using until you can lift them with control. Using momentum and swinging your weights can cause injury, and it's also cheating your muscles.
- **Use full** range of motion. Each exercise has it's own range of motion, and you want to perform each exercise throughout its full range, without locking the joints. For example, in a biceps curl, you want to lower the weight all the way down without losing tension on the muscle or locking the joints. In the upward motion, lift the weights as high as you can without moving the elbows.

You'll find a variety of detailed exercises and workouts in the following chapters, but the following is an example of a typical beginner workout that follows the basic guidelines set out by the ACSM. The sets, reps, and weights listed are only suggestions and may need to be adjusted according to your fitness level.

TOTAL BODY FOR BEGINNERS

Exercise	Sets/Reps	Suggested Weight
Chest press machine	1 x 12	20 pounds
Lat pull-down machine	1 x 12	40 pounds
Overhead press	1 x 12	5–8-pound dumbbells
Biceps curls	1 x 12	8–10-pound dumbbells
Triceps kickbacks	1 x 12	5–8-pound dumbbells
Leg-press machine	1 x 12	20–50 pounds
Lunges	1 x 12	0–8-pound dumbbells
Calf raises	1 x 12	0–10-pound dumbbells
Ab crunches	1 x 12	
Back extensions	1 x 12	

TOOLS YOU NEED

▶ Setting up your own strength-training workouts can be confusing and overwhelming, but there is no perfect program you should be doing. Any strength-training program will work as long as you're challenging your muscles and following the basic principles of strength training. For some ideas on how to get started, visit my Workout Central, which includes a variety of workouts for all fitness levels: http://about.com/exercise/workoutcenter.

Functional Strength Training

Throughout this chapter, you've learned the ins and outs of structured strength training. But there's one other area that's getting more and more popular: functional strength training. In previous chapters, we've talked about setting functional goals, and one way to do that is to approach strength training as something to help you function better. This might be a good choice if you're not quite ready for all-out strength training with heavy weights but you have some improvements you could make with your strength and endurance. In fact, many seniors and overweight and sedentary people begin strength training in this way, only to move on to more vigorous practice as they get stronger.

Functional strength training is exactly what it sounds like: exercises you do to help you function better in life. With this approach, you may not be as focused on using lots of equipment or keeping track of reps and sets. What you're concerned with is mimicking daily movements with focus, concentration and, often, with some added resistance to make your body stronger for what you need to do.

Some examples of functional strength training might include:

- Performing squats in order to improve your ability to get up and down from a chair
- Doing step-ups to help strengthen the legs and make it easier to go up stairs or step up onto curbs while keeping your balance
- Strengthening the abs and back with rotation or bending movements to make gardening or yard work tasks easier
- Doing flexibility and balance exercises to build strength in the stability muscles and connective tissues of the body

Working with a personal trainer is a great way to get insight into the types of exercises you can do to perform your daily tasks with ease. It's important to know what you can safely do, so you should always check with your doctor or an expert if you have specific injuries, illnesses, or conditions you're managing. More details about different types of functional training are also discussed in Chapter 15.

Get Linked

The following resources on my **About.com** *Exercise site will educate you about how to make your strength-training workouts effective, efficient, and challenging.*

EFFECTIVE STRENGTH TRAINING WORKOUTS

Machines and free weights are both great choices for strength training, but there are some machine exercises that you may want to skip in favor of more efficient moves. This article lists some of my least favorite machine exercises and offers alternative moves to help you engage more muscle groups and get more out of your workouts.

 http://about.com/exercise/effectiveworkouts

SETTING UP A STRENGTH TRAINING ROUTINE

There are a number of options for setting up an effective strength-training program, whether you're a beginner or an advanced exerciser. This article details a few popular ways to schedule a strength routine and includes sample workouts to give you some ideas of exercises you can do.

 http://about.com/exercise/strengthroutine

HOW TO GAIN MUSCLE

If your goal is to build muscle, you'll have to work just as hard as a person who wants to lose weight. Building muscle requires careful attention to quality strength-training workouts as well as getting enough calories to fuel your body and add lean muscle tissue. This article describes the basics of building muscle.

 http://about.com/exercise/gainmuscle

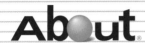

Chapter 6

Strength-Training Exercises

Basic Equipment You'll Need

The following pages detail some of the standard strength-training exercises that target the major muscles of the upper and lower body. Though not every exercise is included, the moves listed will provide a basic foundation for building a strong, fit body.

Most of the exercises involve basic strength-training equipment such as dumbbells, an exercise ball, and a bench or step, but feel free to use any type of resistance or other equipment you have available. If you don't have a ball or a weight bench, feel free to do the exercises on the floor, and if you feel you need extra support for the supine exercises, place a rolled-up towel under your hips for added back support. Your choices for types of resistance include:

- Free weights such as dumbbells or barbells
- Resistance tubes or bands

- Fixed-weight machines
- Cable or free-motion machines
- Body weight

Many exercises will also include a list of variations as well as modifications to fit different fitness levels and equipment types. When you've mastered an exercise, feel free to add intensity by increasing weights or trying more challenging variations.

Just be sure to raise the intensity of the exercises only a little at a time. If you increase weight or resistance too quickly, you could end up with an injury. Remember that you should challenge yourself as you feel ready, but pain is an indication that something could be going wrong. And if you get hurt, you'll have to discontinue most or all exercise to allow yourself time to heal!

When doing your workout, wear comfortable, loose-fitting clothing and supportive shoes and make sure you warm up before each workout with light cardio or light versions of each strength-training exercise. Be sure to modify any move that is uncomfortable to you or to skip any exercises that cause pain or discomfort.

Don't worry that you won't be getting a complete workout if you don't do every single exercise shown in this book. In fact, it's best not to exhaust every muscle group during your workouts. Even if you have a challenging goal you're trying to achieve, your body still needs at least some time to rest in between exercise.

ELSEWHERE ON THE WEB

▶ There are so many exercises you can do that it's hard to know where to start. The great thing about strength training is that there are standard moves for each muscle group, and once you learn those, most other exercises are just variations of those basic moves. For an amazing list of strength-training, stretching, Pilates, and cardio exercises, visit the Exercise Database at www .exercisedb.com.

Chest

Your chest includes some of the larger muscles of the upper body and is made up of the pectoralis major and pectoralis minor. The pectoralis major is the larger muscle in the chest and has two parts: the clavicular head (or the upper chest) and the sternal head (the lower part of the chest). It goes from the collarbone to the sternum and helps in flexion, extension, adduction, and rotation of the shoulder.

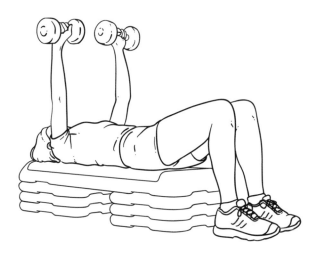

Fig. 6-1

Chest Press with Dumbbells on Step or Bench Fig. 6-1 Begin by lying on the bench and push the weights straight up over the chest without locking the elbows. Bend the elbows and lower the weights until elbows are at about 90 degrees (like a goal post) or just slightly below the chest. Push the weights back up and repeat for 1 to 3 sets of 8 to 12 reps. For variations, do this move on a ball, using a barbell, or on an incline.

Chest Fly with Dumbbells Fig. 6-2
Begin by lying down on the bench holding
the weights over the chest, elbows slightly
bent and pointing out to the sides. Lower
the arms down to the sides to about chest
level keeping the elbows in a fixed position. Bring the weights back together over
the chest in a hugging motion (think of
hugging a tree) until the weights are close
together, and repeat.

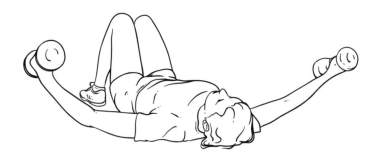

Fig. 6-2

Chest Press with Resistance Tube
Fig. 6-3 Secure the tube to a sturdy object
behind you and hold the handles in each
hand as you sit or stand. Begin the move
with the elbows bent and parallel to the
floor and keep tension on the band as you
press the arms out and in. Repeat for 1 to
3 sets of 8 to 12 reps.

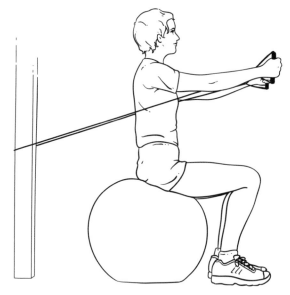

Fig. 6-3

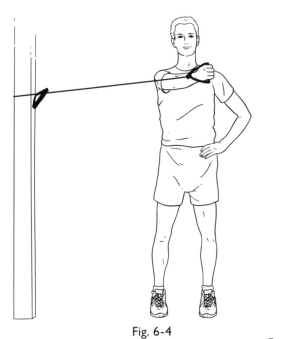

Fig. 6-4

One-Armed Fly with Tube Fig. 6-4
Secure one end of the tube to a sturdy
object and hold the other end in the right
hand. Take a few steps to the side until
there's tension on the band and, keeping
the elbow slightly bent, contract the chest
to bring the arm toward the middle of the
chest, repeating for 1 to 3 sets of 8 to 12
reps.

Push-ups on the Ball Fig. 6-5 Begin
by lying facedown with the ball positioned
under the thighs or shins. Place the hands
on the floor at chest level and slightly wider
than shoulder width. Bend the elbows and
lower down into a push-up, keeping the
back and legs straight. Push the body back
up without locking the elbows and repeat
for 1 to 3 sets of 8 to 12 reps. For variations, roll farther out on the ball or do this
move on the knees or toes.

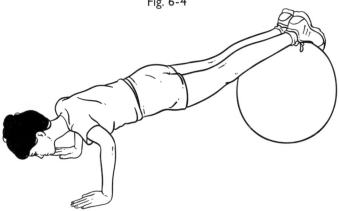

Fig. 6-5

Chapter 6. Strength-Training Exercises |

Push-ups with Resistance Tube Fig. 6-6
Wrap the tubing around your back, looping either side around your hands to keep tension on the band. Get into push-up position, on the knees or toes, holding either side of the tubing in each hand. Lower into a push-up until elbows are at about 90 degrees, and push back up, allowing the tubing to stretch and add intensity to the exercise. Repeat for 1 to 3 sets of 8 to 12 reps.

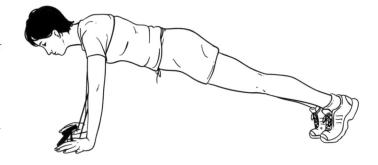

Fig. 6-6

Back

The back is another large muscle group in the upper body and is made up of several muscles. The latissimus dorsi muscles (or lats) are on each side of your back and aid in extension, rotation, and adducting the arms. The erector spinae (lower back) is made up of three muscles that run the length of your back from your neck to your glutes, and flexes, extends, and rotates the upper body. The rhomboids (also know as posture muscles) are in the upper back between the shoulder blades and help in elevation, retraction, and rotation of the shoulder blades. The trapezius muscles in the upper back help move the shoulder blades through various motions as well as extending and rotating the head and neck.

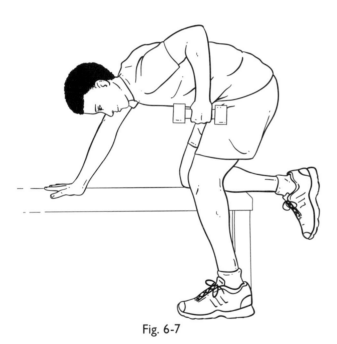

Fig. 6-7

Bent-Over Row Fig. 6-7 Begin by positioning yourself on the side of the bench with right knee and hand resting on it for support. Keep the back flat and the abs contracted. Holding a weight extended with the left hand, contract the back as you pull the elbow up in a rowing motion until it's just above the torso. Lower the weight and extend the arm without locking the joint, and repeat for 1 to 3 sets of 8 to 12 reps.

Bent-Over Row with Resistance Tube Fig. 6-8 Place the tube under both feet and grab the handles in both hands, wrapping the tubing several times to add tension if needed. Bend forward at the waist until the back is flat and parallel to the floor and bend the elbows, bringing them up to torso level as you squeeze the back. Lower and repeat for 1 to 3 sets of 8 to 12 reps.

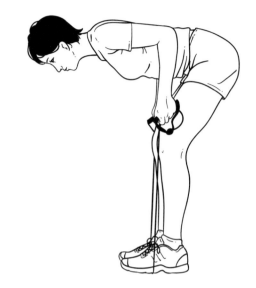

Fig. 6-8

Dumbbell Pullover Fig. 6-9 Lie down on a bench or step and hold a dumbbell in both hands with the arms straight up over the chest. Keeping the elbows slightly bent, slowly lower the arms down behind you until your arms reach the ears or as low as your flexibility allows. Contract the back to pull the arms back up, and repeat for 1 to 3 sets of 8 to 12 reps. If you have shoulder problems, skip this exercise.

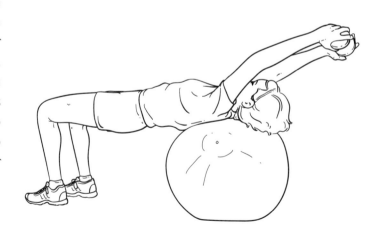

Fig. 6-9

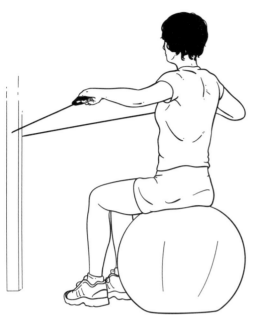

Fig. 6-10

Seated Row with Resistance Tube

Fig. 6-10 Secure the tube around a sturdy object and sit or stand far enough away that there's tension on the tube. Holding handles in each hand, begin with the arms straight out in front and parallel to the floor. Pull the elbows back toward the torso, squeezing the shoulder blades together and keeping the forearms parallel to the ground. Return to starting position and repeat for 1 to 3 sets of 8 to 12 reps.

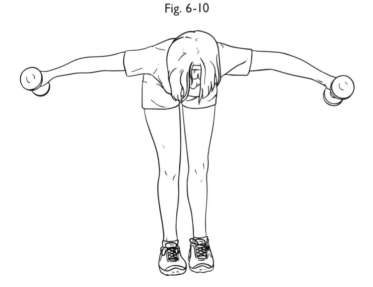

Fig. 6-11

Bent-Over Reverse Fly Fig. 6-11 In a standing position, bend forward at the waist with abs in and back flat, weights hanging down with palms facing each other. With elbows slightly bent and fixed, squeeze the shoulder blades together as you lift the arms out to the sides to shoulder level. Lower down and repeat.

If I don't have equipment, can I still get an effective workout?

▶ If you want to build strength and muscle, you'll eventually need to add resistance during your workouts. But if you're just starting out or are on a tight budget, you can still get a challenging workout by doing bodyweight exercises. To make them more intense, simply slow down the moves (for example, during a squat, take four seconds to lower down and push back up) and do more repetitions.

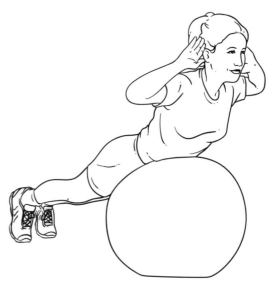

Fig. 6-12

Back Extension on the Ball Fig. 6-12 Lie facedown with the ball positioned under the hips and stomach and the legs out, resting on the toes. You can place your hands behind the head or under the chin. Keeping the head in a neutral position, lift the head and shoulders up by contracting the muscles of the lower back. Continue lifting until the back is straight; lower and repeat for 1 to 3 sets of 8 to 12 reps. For variations, you can do this move on the floor or on a back-extension apparatus.

Shoulders

The muscles of the shoulder, or the deltoids, have three different areas: the anterior (front), lateral (side), and posterior (rear). Though it's all one muscle, each part of the shoulder works a bit differently from the other. The front of the deltoid flexes and rotates the arm inward, the side deltoid abducts the arm, and the rear deltoid extends and rotates the arm outward.

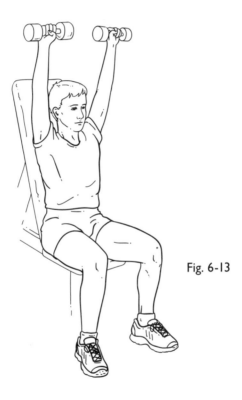

Fig. 6-13

Overhead Press Fig. 6-13 In a seated or standing position, begin with arms at shoulder height, elbows bent, and palms facing out. Keeping abs contracted and back straight, push the weights up over the head until your arms are extended but not locked. Lower back to starting position and repeat for 1 to 3 sets of 8 to 12 reps. For a variation, do this exercise with a resistance tube positioned under your feet.

Lateral Raise Fig. 6-14 Begin with feet about hip-width apart, knees slightly bent, and weights in front with palms facing each other. With elbows fixed and slightly bent, lift the arms up to shoulder level until they're parallel to the floor, squeezing the shoulders. Lower back to starting position and repeat for 1 to 3 sets of 8 to 12 reps. For a variation, do this with a resistance tube.

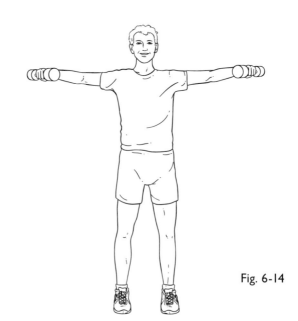

Fig. 6-14

Front Raise Fig. 6-15 Begin in a standing position holding light dumbbells in front of the thighs. Keeping the abs contracted, slowly lift the arms straight up to shoulder level. To avoid swinging the weights, take one foot back in a split stance. Continue lifting and lowering for 1 to 3 sets of 8 to 12 reps.

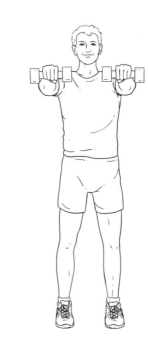

Fig. 6-15

Arms

The major muscles of the arms include the biceps, triceps, and forearms. The biceps actually have two parts, a long head and a short head and are responsible for flexing the elbow and supination of the forearm. The triceps have three parts—the long head, lateral head, and short head—and are responsible for extending the elbow. The muscles of the forearms include the brachioradialis as well as a number of muscles designed to flex and extend the wrist as well as rotate the forearm.

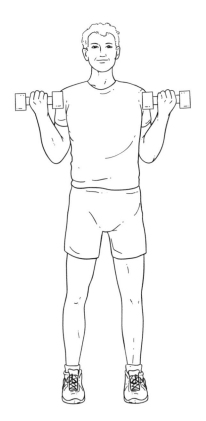

Fig. 6-16

Biceps Curls Fig. 6-16 Begin with feet about hip-width apart and weights in front of the thighs, palms facing out. Contract the biceps muscles and bend the elbows, bringing the weights toward the shoulders. Lower the weight without locking the elbow joint or losing tension on the muscle and repeat for 1 to 3 sets of 8 to 12 reps. For a variation, turn the palms in for a hammer curl or do this exercise with a barbell or resistance tube.

Concentration Curls Fig. 6-17 Sit on a ball or bench and prop the right elbow against the inside of the right thigh, with the weight hanging down. Using the thigh for leverage, bend the elbow and bring the weight up toward the shoulder, squeezing the bicep. Repeat for 1 to 3 sets of 8 to 12 reps.

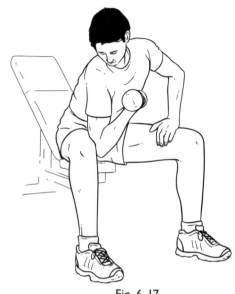

Fig. 6-17

Triceps Kickbacks Fig. 6-18 Stand in a split stance with right leg forward and left leg back, right hand resting on the thigh or a chair for support. Holding a weight in the left hand, bend forward at the waist and bring the elbow up to torso level, arm bent. Straighten the arm, pressing the weight back until the arm is fully extended but not locked. Lower and repeat for 1 to 3 sets of 8 to 12 reps.

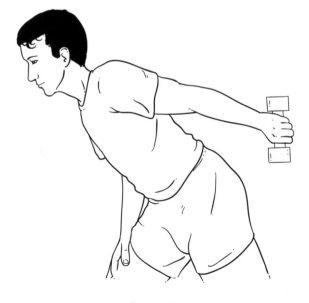

Fig. 6-18

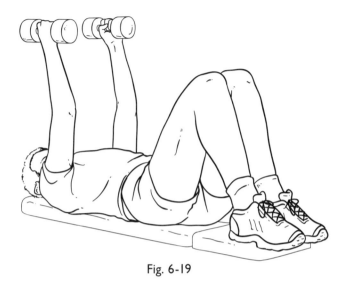

Fig. 6-19

Lying Triceps Extensions Fig. 6-19 Lie on the floor or on a bench and hold weights in both hands. Bring the arms straight up over the chest with palms facing each other and bend the elbows, bringing the weights down next to the ears. Squeeze the triceps to lift the arms back up, and repeat for 1 to 3 sets of 8 to 12 reps.

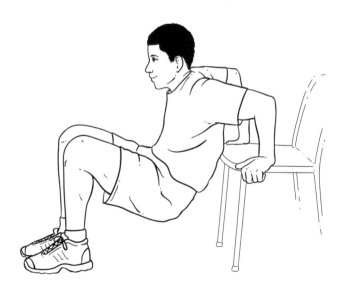

Fig. 6-20

Triceps Dips Fig. 6-20 Begin by sitting on a chair or step and place the hands beside the hips. Lift up onto your hands and bring the hips just in front of the chair. Bend the elbows and lower the body down until the elbows are at about 90 degrees, keeping the shoulders down and away from the ears. Squeeze the triceps to push back up to starting position, repeating for 1 to 3 sets of 8 to 12 reps. For added intensity, move the legs farther out in front of you.

Lower Body

The lower body includes the largest muscles in the body, the glutes, as well as other large muscle complexes like the quads, hamstrings, and calves. These muscles are involved in almost every move you make each day and will burn the most calories in both cardio and strength-training exercises.

Ball Squats Fig. 6-21 Position the ball against a wall so that it's just behind the lower back. Lean against the ball and walk the feet out slightly, keeping them about hip-width apart. Contract the abs and slowly lower into a squat by bending the knees and taking the glutes out behind you, keeping the knees behind the toes. Go down as low as you can or until the upper thighs are parallel to the floor, and push into the heels to come back up. Repeat for 1 to 3 sets of 8 to 12 reps. For variations, hold weights or do this exercise without the ball and with weights or a barbell for an added challenge.

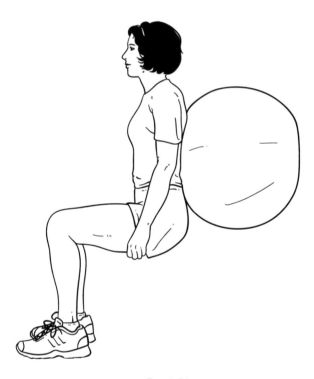

Fig. 6-21

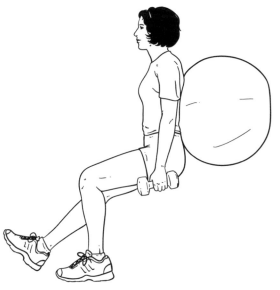

One-Legged Squats Fig. 6-22 Position the ball behind the lower back and bring the left leg in front of the body, lifting the right leg slightly off the floor. Bend the left knee and lower into a slight squat, touching the right foot down for balance if needed. Push into the heel to come back up, and repeat for 1 to 3 sets of 8 to 12 reps. To make this move easier, lightly rest the non-working foot on the floor throughout the movement.

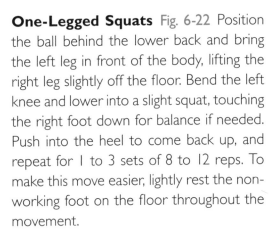

Fig. 6-22

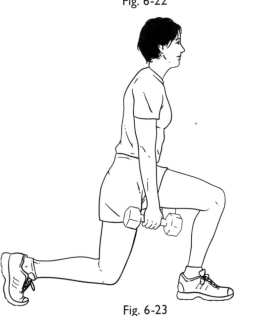

Lunges Fig. 6-23 Stand in a split stance with feet about two or more feet apart. Lower into a lunge by bending both knees, dropping the back knee straight down toward the floor. Lunge as low as you can without touching the floor. Push into the floor to come back to starting position and repeat for 1 to 3 sets of 8 to 12 reps before switching sides. For variations, you can perform walking lunges or step backward or to the side. To add intensity, hold weights or use a barbell.

Fig. 6-23

Deadlifts Fig. 6-24 Begin with feet about shoulder width apart, knees fixed but slightly bent, weights resting in front of the thighs. Keeping the shoulders back, abs in, and the back straight or slightly arched, tip from the hips and lower the weights down until you feel a stretch in the hamstrings or until you feel your back begin to round. Shift the weight back into the heels slightly and squeeze the glutes to come up; repeat for 1 to 3 sets of 8 to 12 reps.

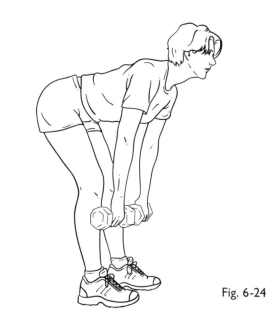

Fig. 6-24

One-Legged Deadlifts Fig. 6-25 Begin by holding weights in front of the thighs and bring the left leg out behind you with the toe resting lightly on the floor. Keeping the shoulders back and the abs contracted, bend from the hips and lower the weights down toward the floor. Squeeze the glutes to come up and repeat for 1 to 3 sets of 8 to 12 reps before switching sides. For variations, lift the nonworking leg completely off the floor or rest it on a ball or step.

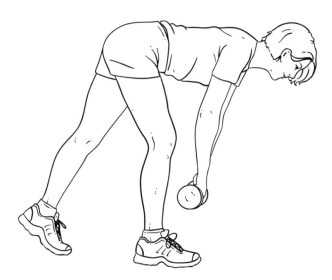

Fig. 6-25

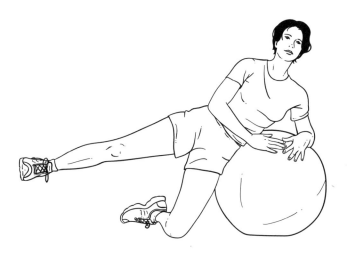

Leg Lifts on the Ball Fig. 6-26 Lie with your left side resting on the ball with the left knee on the floor for support. Keeping the hips stacked and the torso straight, flex the right foot and slowly lift it a few inches off the floor. Lower the leg without touching the floor and repeat for 1 to 3 sets of 8 to 12 reps. To add intensity, use light to medium ankle weights on the working leg.

Fig. 6-26

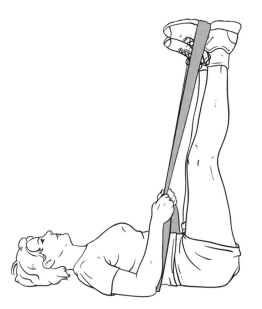

Crisscross Outer Thigh Fig. 6-27 Lie on the floor and loop the tube around both feet. Lift the legs straight up, keeping a slight bend in the knees if needed. Cross the tube in front of you and grab the handles in opposite hands, pulling tight on the tube to add tension. Keeping the knees straight and the feet flexed, open the legs out to either side, squeezing the glutes. Come back to starting position and repeat for 1 to 3 sets of 8 to 12 reps.

Fig. 6-27

Inner Thigh Ball Squeeze Fig. 6-28
Lie on the floor and lift the legs, placing
the ball between the knees. Keeping the
abs contracted and the lower back pressed
into the floor, squeeze the ball and release
slightly, keeping tension on the ball throughout the movement. Repeat for 1 to 3 sets
of 8 to 12 reps. To make this move easier,
rest the legs on the floor and sit back onto
your forearms.

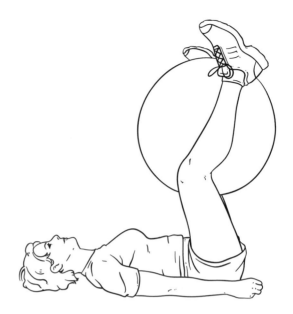

Fig. 6-28

Hamstring Rolls on the Ball Fig. 6-29
Lie on the floor and place the heels on
the ball. Lift the hips off the floor until the
body is in a straight line, and squeeze
the hamstrings to roll the ball in toward
the glutes. Roll the ball out and repeat for
1 to 3 sets of 8 to 12 reps, keeping the hips
lifted throughout the movement. To make
this move easier, rest the hips on the floor
during each rep. To make it harder, do it
one leg at a time.

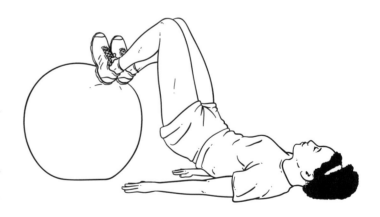

Fig. 6-29

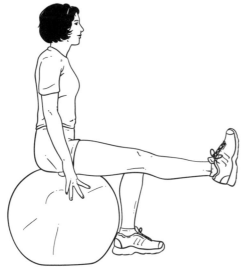

Fig. 6-30

Leg Extensions Fig. 6-30 Sit on a ball or chair with the abs in, back straight, and shoulders back. Keeping the knees together and at the same level, straighten the right leg, squeezing the quads. Lower and repeat for 1 to 3 sets of 8 to 12 reps before switching to the other leg. For more difficulty, add ankle weights to this exercise.

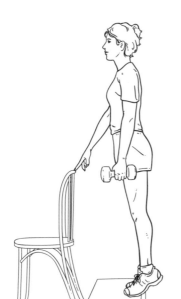

Fig. 6-31

Calf Raises Fig. 6-31 Stand on the floor and hold onto a wall or chair for balance if needed. Lift up onto your toes as high as you can, repeating for 1 to 3 sets of 8 to 12 reps. For a variation, do this move on a step or platform to get more range of motion. You can also hold on to weights for added intensity. (These two variations are shown in Figure 6-31.)

Core

The term *core* is a broad term covering all the muscles in the abs, pelvis, and back. These muscles include (but aren't limited to) the rectus abdominis (the "six-pack" muscles), the internal and external obliques, the transverse abdominis, and the muscles of the hips and lower back. Having a strong core means more than just working the abs; it means doing a variety of dynamic exercises to strengthen the torso, which protects your back from injury and gives you a strong center for all your activities and exercises.

Crunches on the Ball Fig. 6-32 Lie faceup with the ball positioned under the mid-lower back, knees bent and hands behind the head or crossed over the chest. Contract the abs to lift the head and shoulders up into a slight C shape, keeping the chin tucked. Lower back down, keeping tension on the abs, and repeat for 1 to 3 sets of 8 to 16 reps. You can also do this move on the floor for a modified version.

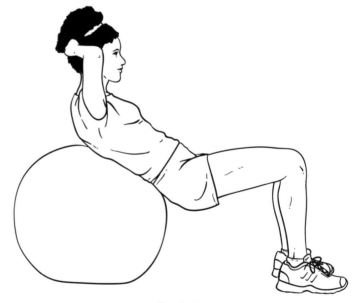

Fig. 6-32

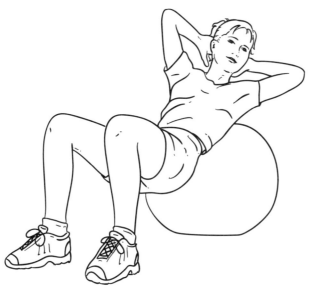

Oblique Crunch on the Ball Fig. 6-33
Lie on your back on the ball, with knees bent and hands gently cradling the head. Contract the abs and lift the shoulders off the ball; then rotate the torso, reaching the right shoulder toward the left knee. Lower and repeat for 1 to 3 sets of 8 to 16 reps before switching sides. Do this move on the floor for a modified version.

Fig. 6-33

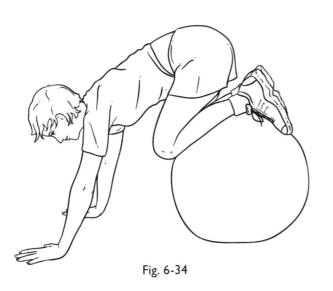

Knee Tucks on the Ball Fig. 6-34
Kneeling in front of the ball, gently roll forward into a push-up position, with the ball positioned under the shins. Bend the knees and roll the ball in while contracting the abs, and slowly roll the ball back to starting position. Repeat for 1 to 3 sets of 8 to 12 reps. To make this move harder, bring the body into a pike position with the legs straight instead of tucking the knees.

Fig. 6-34

Reverse Crunches Fig. 6-35 Lie on the floor and gently cradle your head in your hands as you lift the legs straight up, knees slightly bent. Keep the head and shoulders lifted off the floor and contract the lower abs to lift the hips off the floor, sending the feet straight up toward the ceiling. Lower and repeat for 1 to 3 sets of 8 to 16 reps. If this hurts your neck, you can rest your head on the floor. For a variation, do this move with the ball tucked behind your knees.

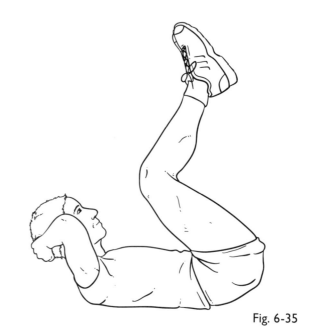

Fig. 6-35

Bicycle Fig. 6-36 Lie on the floor and cradle your head in your hands as you bring the knees in toward the chest. Straighten the left leg out as you rotate the torso to the right, bringing your left elbow toward the right knee. Repeat the move to the other side, alternating for 1 to 3 sets of 8 to 16 reps on each side.

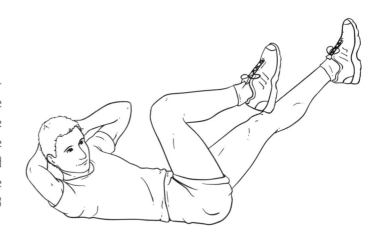

Fig. 6-36

Get Linked

The following resources on my About.com Exercise site offer more information about strength-training exercises and workouts for a variety of goals and fitness levels.

STRENGTH TRAINING AND SPECIALTY WORKOUTS

Learning which exercises work the different muscles of the body can be confusing. This index lists a variety of strength-training workouts for the lower body, upper body, abs, and more, to help you learn more about exercises you can do for various parts of your body.

http://about.com/exercise/workouts

ABS

It's important to work your abs for a strong, fit body, but you don't necessarily need to work them every day. In fact, there are a variety of ways to work your abs without doing a single crunch. Learn more by visiting this page for FAQs, articles, and workout ideas for your abs.

http://about.com/exercise/abs

BUTT, HIPS, AND THIGHS

Working the lower body is essential for burning calories and building strong muscles, but you may wonder what exercises you should do for lean legs. This index lists a variety of workouts, FAQs, and articles to help you navigate the confusing world of strength training and weight loss for the lower body.

http://about.com/exercise/butthipsthighs

The **ABOUT.com** *Guide to* **Getting in Shape**

Chapter 7

Flexibility and Mind/Body Exercise

Why You Need to Stretch

While most people wouldn't argue that being flexible is important, stretching is the one area of fitness that is often overlooked. We focus so much on cardio and strength training that flexibility training often takes a backseat to everything else. Why waste time and energy on something that isn't going to burn a lot of calories or make you stronger? But being flexible and stretching on a regular basis is important for a number of reasons:

- It helps relax the muscles you've been working.
- It increases your range of motion.
- It helps improve balance and coordination.
- It can help protect the body from injuries during certain activities.
- It feels good and leaves you feeling more relaxed.

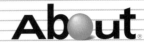

▶ **Tight muscles can lead to a number of aches and pains in the body and are often caused by bad posture and hours of sitting. Some common problems with posture include rounded shoulders, which can lead to tightness in the chest, and a forward head, which can strain the neck and upper back. How's your posture? Find out by taking a few simple tests in my article "Strengthen Your Core," at http://about.com/ exercise/core. There you'll find simple tips for improving your posture.**

A simple definition of *flexibility* is the range of motion within a joint and along a variety of planes of movement. How your joints move depend on a number of factors that we often can't control, like our genes or the structure of the joints and connective tissues. But one factor we can control is how flexible our muscles are, and that flexibility is what allows us to move through different activities smoothly and gracefully.

People often wonder about the best time to stretch. Should you stretch before your workout, after, or both? Science has found that stretching before a workout won't necessarily protect you from injury, as was once thought, and that too much stretching may actually cause injuries in some cases. One common reason for injuries is stretching muscles that are cold and tight, which can cause muscle tears or strains. Whether you stretch before or after your workout, you'll want to make sure your muscles are warm, either after a warm-up or after exercise.

I usually recommend that my clients stretch after their workouts, especially during cardio exercise, because it saves time. Rather than stopping to stretch after your warm-up, which can cause your heart rate to drop, you may want to stretch after the cooldown, when muscles are warm and pliable and you don't have to worry about keeping your heart rate up anymore.

When stretching, you want to follow a few simple rules to avoid injury and get the most out of the exercises:

- As mentioned previously, make sure your muscles are warm before you stretch, either with exercise or after a hot bath or shower.
- Stretches should be gentle and slow to allow your muscles time to relax into the exercises.

- Don't bounce when performing static stretches; when you bounce or stretch too far, your muscles may contract to protect themselves, and this can lead to injuries and pain.
- When doing static stretches, hold them for about ten to thirty seconds, and repeat each stretch one to three times.
- Only stretch as far as you comfortably can; you shouldn't feel pain during flexibility exercises.

There are different ways to stretch the body, but the most common are passive (or static), dynamic, and active stretches. Passive or static stretching is the most popular way to stretch, involving holding each stretch for a specific period of time. Dynamic stretching involves warming up the body for specific activities with exercises like arm swings, leg swings, or flexing and extending the joints. Active stretching (also called active isolated stretching [AIS]) involves stretching a muscle by contracting the opposite muscle. To see how these different stretches work, think of a hamstring stretch. A static hamstring stretch would involve taking one leg out and bending forward to feel a stretch in the back of the leg. A dynamic stretch for the hamstring would be lightly swinging the leg back and forth. An active stretch would involve lifting the leg straight up as high as you can and holding it there, allowing the quad to contract as the hamstring stretches.

Basic Stretches for Each Muscle Group

The following exercises show a few standard static stretches that can be used to stretch the muscles you've worked during exercise. Be sure to work within your own range of motion, to a point that's comfortable for your body.

WHAT'S HOT

▶ Originally used to rehabilitate patients after surgery, active isolated stretching (AIS) is becoming more mainstream as we look for more functional ways to increase flexibility. In AIS, you contract one muscle while stretching the opposing muscle, and experts believe this allows a deeper, more complete stretch. Instead of holding a static stretch, AIS stretches are held for one or two seconds and repeated for several reps. For more, check out Jay Blahnik's excellent book, *Full-Body Flexibility*.

Hamstring Stretch Fig. 7-1

1. Lie down with knees bent and bring the right knee in toward the chest, holding the leg just behind the knee.
2. Straighten the right leg and gently pull it toward you until you feel a stretch in the hamstring; bend the knee to make the move more comfortable if you're tight.
3. Hold the stretch for 10 to 30 seconds and switch legs.

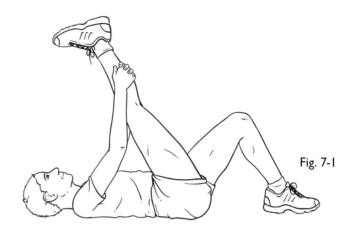

Fig. 7-1

Quad Stretch Fig. 7-2

1. Lie on your left side, hips stacked, and bend the right knee, bringing the foot toward the glutes.
2. Hold on to the foot with the right hand and keep the knees level as you gently pull the foot in, feeling a stretch in the front of the thigh.
3. Hold the stretch for 10 to 30 seconds, gently pushing the right hip forward for a deeper stretch. Repeat on the other side.

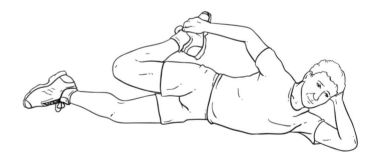

Fig. 7-2

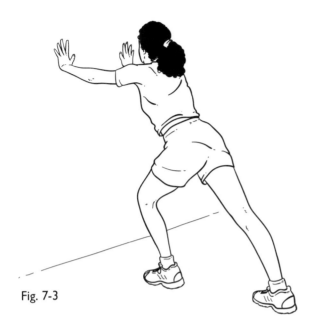

Fig. 7-3

Calf Stretch Fig. 7-3

1. Place hands on a wall in front of you and extend the right leg back, knee straight but not locked.
2. Press the right heel toward the floor until you feel a gentle stretch in the calf muscle.
3. Hold for 10 to 30 seconds and switch sides.

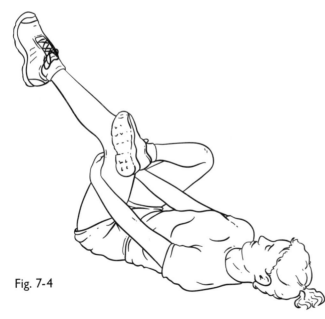

Fig. 7-4

Hip Stretch Fig. 7-4

1. Lie on the floor with knees bent and cross the right foot over the left knee.
2. Reach forward to grasp the left thigh with both hands, gently pulling it toward the chest as you gently push the right knee back, feeling the stretch in your right hip and glute.
3. Hold for 10 to 30 seconds and repeat on the other leg.

Chest Stretch Fig. 7-5

1. While standing, place the hands behind the head, elbows out to the sides.
2. Gently pull the elbows back behind the ears until you feel a stretch across the chest.
3. Hold for 10 to 30 seconds and repeat.

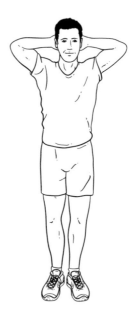

Fig. 7-5

Shoulder Stretch Fig. 7-6

1. While standing, reach the right arm straight across the body and over the chest.
2. Place the left hand on the right elbow and gently pull the arm across the body while dropping the right shoulder down.
3. Hold for 10 to 30 seconds and repeat with the other arm.

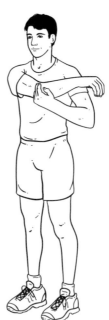

Fig. 7-6

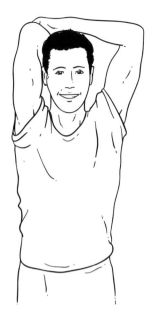

Fig. 7-7

ASK YOUR GUIDE

How do I know if I need to be more flexible?

▶ How flexible you need to be is really based on whether you can accomplish what you need to without pain or tightness. For example, if you can't bend over without feeling pain or pulling in your back or hamstrings, that may make you more susceptible to back injuries. Pay attention to areas that feel tight or tender throughout the day and make a point to stretch those areas whenever you can.

Triceps Stretch Fig. 7-7

1. Stretch the right arm straight up overhead next to the ear and bend the arm, taking the forearm behind the head or back behind you.
2. Place the left hand on the right elbow and gently pull the arm toward your head until you feel a stretch in the back of the arm.
3. Hold for 10 to 30 seconds and repeat with the other arm.

▶ Yoga has become a popular activity, but a new and growing trend involves yoga classes that focus on specific goals such as lower-back pain, gaining strength, and getting better at sports like golf and tennis. These kinds of classes may offer a greater appeal, providing new ways to incorporate yoga in a functional way. My Yoga Fusion Workout (http://about.com/exercise/yoga fusion) offers a blend of yoga moves with resistance bands to add intensity and increase muscular endurance.

Understanding Yoga

If you're looking for balance, flexibility, and relaxation, yoga is an excellent choice, combing all of these elements into poses and postures that flow together, with an emphasis on breathing. The word *yoga* means "union" and describes the union among the body, mind, and spirit. This kind of mindful exercise, or what some call a moving meditation, requires you to focus your attention inward and be present in the moment. While it doesn't typically offer the calorie burn of cardio or the strength gains of resistance training, yoga is a great complement to these other disciplines, giving you a chance to slow down, stretch the body, and let go of tension and stress.

In the past few years, scientists have been studying yoga in a variety of ways and have found that the benefits of yoga include:

● Decreased blood pressure
● Decreased stress, anxiety, depression, and insomnia
● Increased flexibility, strength, balance, and coordination
● Improved posture
● Increased relaxation and a sense of well-being

There are several branches of yoga, each of which has its own focus and purpose, but the most popular branch is hatha yoga. Hatha yoga involves moving through a wide range of postures that can be done standing, seated, lying on the floor, and even upside down. The idea is to move through the poses and postures while following a breathing pattern, increasing the difficulty of the moves as you get stronger and more flexible. If you start a yoga practice, you'll find there are various types of yoga, each a little different from the other:

● **Iyengar yoga** places an emphasis on body alignment along with the breath; in this type of yoga, you might spend longer periods of time holding each pose and using props (such as blocks or straps) to help you get into proper alignment.

- **Restorative yoga** is a gentle form of yoga and great for beginners; this type of yoga focuses on simple, often supported poses, with an emphasis on relaxing and releasing stress.
- **Ashtanga yoga**, also known as power yoga, tends to be fast-paced and more intense than other types of yoga, with an emphasis on strength, flexibility, and stamina.
- **Bikram yoga**, also called hot yoga, is practiced in a hot room, with temperatures ranging from 95 to 100 degrees. The classes are usually ninety minutes long and more intense and vigorous than in other forms of yoga.

You don't have to know the details of every type of yoga, but it's helpful to know the basics so you know what you're getting into, whether you're taking a class or trying your own practice at home.

The best thing about yoga is that you can practice it anywhere, without any special equipment. But to get the most out of your practice, you might take classes at a yoga studio or health club where an experienced instructor can help you do each pose correctly. Some instructors even offer one-on-one sessions, which is a good choice if you want to get a deeper understanding of each pose.

If taking a class isn't an option, there are a number of yoga DVDs and books available for every fitness level and interest at bookstores and discount stores.

Yoga Exercises

The following workout offers some basic yoga poses designed to stretch and strengthen the body. You can use these examples to practice some of the standard moves you might see in a typical yoga class or workout. For in-depth instructions for each pose, visit our Yoga Guide, Ann Pizer, at About.com: http://yoga.about.com.

ELSEWHERE ON THE WEB

▶ One of the most important parts of a yoga practice is breathing. During yoga, you'll use your breath in different ways to bring the poses to life and focus your attention on what you're doing. To help you learn more about the proper way to breathe in yoga, Ann Pizer, About.com's Yoga Guide, describes a variety of techniques in her Yoga Breathing Exercises index, at http://about.com/yoga/breathing.

Cat and Camel Fig. 7-8 Start on all fours with hands under shoulders and knees under hips. Exhale and drop the head while rounding the back up toward the ceiling, abs tight. Then inhale and look up while tilting the hips up toward the ceiling. Continue moving through each pose for 5 or more breaths.

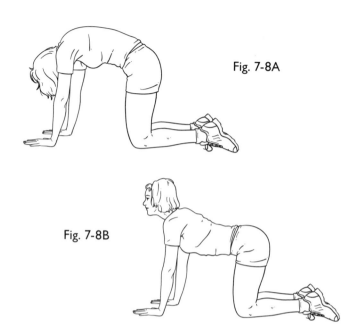

Fig. 7-8A

Fig. 7-8B

Thread the Needle Fig. 7-9 Sit back on the heels and stretch the arms out in front of you. Reach the right arm under the body, palm up, gently stretching the shoulder. Hold for 3 to 5 breaths and repeat on the other side.

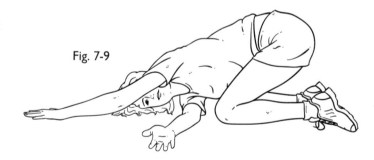

Fig. 7-9

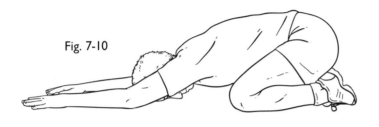

Fig. 7-10

Child's Pose Fig. 7-10 Sit back on the heels with the knees out as you fold forward until your head rests on the mat, arms at your sides. Release the back and hips and hold for 3 to 5 breaths.

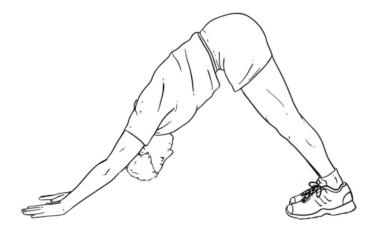

Fig. 7-11

Downward Facing Dog Fig. 7-11 On hands and knees, push the body up into an inverted V shape, pressing into the floor with your hands while pushing heels toward the floor.

Cobra Fig. 7-12 Lying on the floor, place the hands on either side of the chest, elbows bent. Inhale and push through the hands to lift the chest and head off the floor as high as you comfortably can, keeping the shoulders down and relaxed. Hold for 3 to 5 breaths.

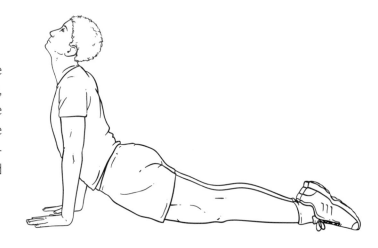

Fig. 7-12

Warrior I Fig. 7-13 Bring the right foot forward and the left leg back, toes out at about 45 degrees, and the heel pressing into the floor. Bend the right knee and square the hips to the front of the room as you bring the arms up overhead, stretching back in a slight backbend. Hold for 3 to 5 breaths.

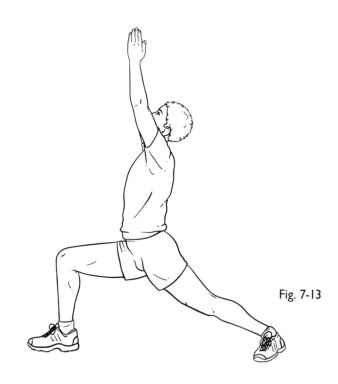

Fig. 7-13

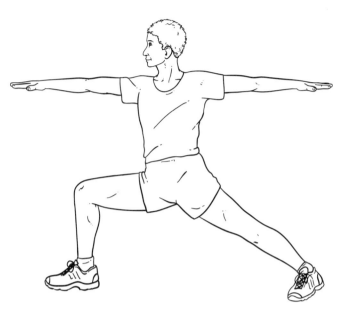

Warrior II Fig. 7-14 From Warrior I, bring the arms down to shoulder level as you turn the body to the side keeping the front knee bent. Gaze out over the hand in front and hold for 3 to 5 breaths.

Fig. 7-14

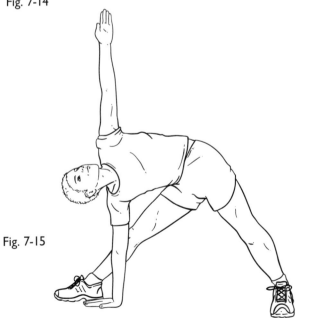

Triangle Pose Fig. 7-15 From Warrior II, straighten the front knee and reach the arm forward, lowering the hand down to the ankle or shin. Reach the other arm straight up to the sky and gaze up at that hand for 3 to 5 breaths.

Fig. 7-15

Tree Pose Fig. 7-16 In a standing position with hands together in a prayer pose, bend the right knee and place the foot on the left calf (easier) or the inside of the left thigh (more advanced). Find your balance and slowly push the hands straight up over the head. Lower and repeat on the other side.

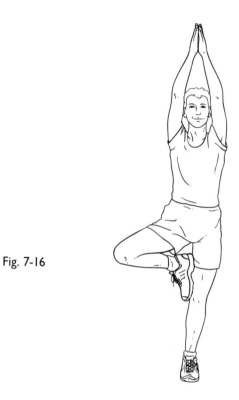

Fig. 7-16

Corpse Pose Fig. 7-17 Lie down with the legs a comfortable distance apart, feet flopped out. Bring the arms out from the body with the palms up and relax the body from head to toe as you breath. Continue for 5 or more minutes, focusing on breathing and relaxing.

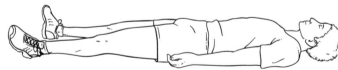

Fig. 7-17

Understanding Pilates

Another popular mind/body activity is Pilates. While many people think Pilates and yoga are the same thing, Pilates actually offers something different from yoga. There are some similarities—both focus on a mind/body connection and both synchronize movement with breath. But the purpose of Pilates, created by Joseph H. Pilates to help rehabilitate injuries, is to create more efficient movement by teaching you how to align your body to minimize undesirable muscle activity. In other words, you learn how to engage the muscles of your pelvis and core (your "powerhouse") to stabilize the body, improve posture, and align the spine. What most people notice when practicing Pilates is that it takes tremendous core strength and is a great way to work your abs, back, hips, and pelvis in different ways.

Like yoga, Pilates isn't a cardio workout, nor is it a strength-training workout, so you still need to do those other activities for fitness and weight loss. But Pilates does offer other benefits such as:

- Better body mechanics
- Improved balance
- Higher level of coordination
- Better strength and flexibility

Pilates also offers that mind/body connection and inner focus often lacking in other types of activities.

There are different types of Pilates workouts available, some based on the original series of exercises created by Joseph Pilates, and others based on the concept of the original Pilates but following different exercises. There are mat classes where you do most exercises on the floor, using your own body weight, and there are other classes that incorporate special equipment (such as the

TOOLS YOU NEED

▸ Many yoga classes involve props such as blocks and straps to provide support for your body as you move through the poses. The exercise ball is one tool you can use during your stretching and yoga workouts to enhance the stretch while providing support so you can do the exercises without straining yourself. My Relaxing Stretch Workout on the ball offers ideas for how to use your ball for different flexibility and yoga exercises. Visit http://about.com/exercise/relaxingstretch.

Reformer), similar to what Joseph Pilates developed in his original workout. Mat classes are the most common and usually the most accessible, offered in studios, gyms, and health clubs. You'll also find plenty of fusion workouts, combining elements of Pilates and yoga together into something called Yogalates.

A typical Pilates class is about forty-five to sixty minutes long and incorporates moves that force you to stabilize the body (using your core and pelvic muscles) as you move through a variety of postures and exercises. It's best to take a class with an experienced and educated instructor, but if that's not an option, there are a number of beginner Pilates videos, such as the Winsor Pilates beginner series, which explain how to do each move with good form and technique.

Pilates Exercises

If you're interested in trying Pilates, your best bet is to work with an experienced instructor who can teach you each exercise and take you through the breathing patterns, which, like yoga, are essential for getting the most out of the exercises. It's important to do Pilates exercises in a certain order and with good form and breathing techniques. The exercises below give you a taste of what Pilates exercises look like and what you can expect when taking a Pilates class, but be sure to work with an expert to learn proper breathing and form.

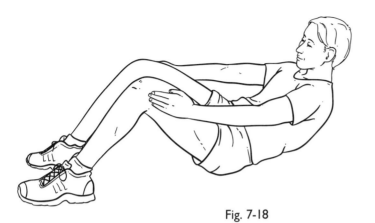

Roll Up Fig. 7-18 Lie down with the legs straight and the arms stretched out over your head. Inhale and lift the arms up to the ceiling and then exhale as you roll up off the mat, one vertebrae at a time. Keep the abs engaged as you exhale and stretch the arms over your legs, keeping a C shape, and then roll back down, feeling each part of your spine make contact with the mat.

Fig. 7-18

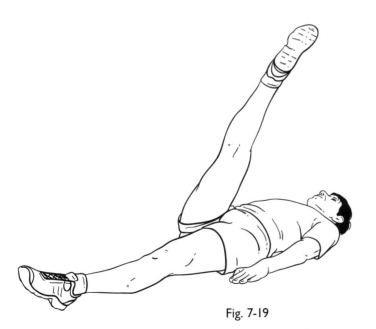

Leg Circles Fig. 7-19 Bring one leg up into the air, slightly bent or straight. Keeping your abs engaged to stabilize the torso and pelvis, make three small circles with the leg clockwise and then counterclockwise. Repeat with the other leg.

Fig. 7-19

Double Leg Stretch Fig. 7-20 Lie down and pull the knees into the chest, with hands resting below the knees. Inhale and contract the abs to lift the shoulders off the floor, then exhale as you reach your arms and legs out in opposite directions, extending through the fingers and toes without arching the back. Come back to start and repeat for 5 to 8 reps. To modify the move, don't fully extend the arms and legs.

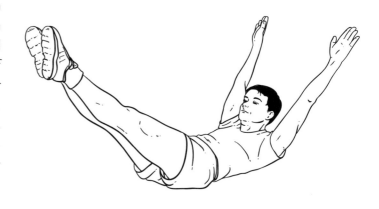

Fig. 7-20

Side Kicks Fig. 7-21 Lie on your right side and bring the legs a bit forward to about 45 degrees. Lift the left leg up slightly and inhale as you swing the leg forward with foot flexed, keeping the torso and hips stable. Exhale and swing the leg back, toes pointed, and repeat for 5 or more reps before switching sides.

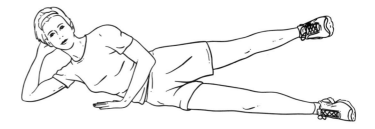

Fig. 7-21

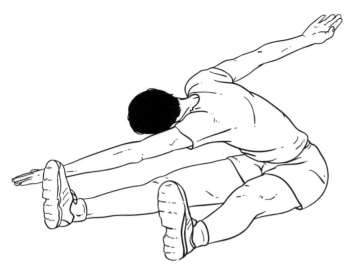

Fig. 7-22

Saw Fig. 7-22 Sit with legs extended wider than shoulders and lift the arms out to the sides, palms down. Inhale and lengthen through the spine, then exhale and rotate to the right, reaching your left hand past your right foot while stretching the other arm behind you. Inhale back to start and repeat to the other side for 6 reps.

Can men do Pilates or is it just for women?

▶ Pilates may seem like an activity for women simply because you'll usually see more women doing Pilates than men. But Pilates is good for everyone, especially men since they tend to be less flexible than women. In fact, there are plenty of male athletes, from basketball players to golfers, who practice Pilates to build a strong, flexible core for better performance.

Get Linked

The following resources on my About.com *Exercise site offer more information about flexibility and mind/body exercises and workouts for a variety of goals and fitness levels.*

STRETCH YOUR LIMITS

This article provides more tips for stretching as well as tools, videos, and books to help you get the most out of your flexibility program.

 http://about.com/exercise/stretching

YOGA AND PILATES-BASED WORKOUTS

These workouts offer some basic yoga and Pilates-type workouts for beginner and intermediate exercisers that focus on core strength, flexibility, and balance.

 http://about.com/exercise/yogapilates

FLEXIBILITY WORKOUTS

These free flexibility workouts are great for all fitness levels and cover a wide range of goals, from becoming more flexible to feeling more relaxed and energized.

 http://about.com/exercise/flexibility

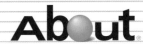

Chapter 8

Workouts to Suit Your Schedule and Goals

Total-Body Strength Workouts by Level

When beginning a strength-training program, it's often best to start with a total-body routine to build a strong foundation and condition your body for more vigorous exercise. One of the benefits of a total-body routine is that you start with fewer exercises, which allows you to perfect your form, learn some of the basic principles of strength training, and build strength and endurance.

Total-body workouts are often easy to follow and tend to be less complicated than split routines, which may be more appealing to beginners. The general rule is to try to get in two to three non-consecutive total-body workouts each week. Make sure you rest at least a day between workouts, but try not to rest too long. Taking too much time can cause you to lose some of the strength and endurance you've gained, so that it's almost like starting all over.

The following total-body workouts range from beginner to intermediate and get progressively more difficult in the length, exercises, sets, and weights for each exercise and workout. Start with a workout that fits your fitness level and goals and adjust the exercises, weights, and/or sets as needed so that you're challenged but not feeling pain.

Total-Body Strength for Beginners The following workout includes exercises targeting the major muscles in the upper and lower body, as well as the abs and lower back. The sets, reps, and weights listed are only guidelines, so modify according to your fitness level. If you've never lifted weights or it's been a long time, start with one set and choose a moderate weight you feel comfortable with. If the workout seems too easy, you can add more sets, more weight, or move on to more difficult workouts. When performing more than one set, rest about 30 to 60 seconds between sets. Before you get started, warm up with a few minutes of light cardio exercise.

TOTAL-BODY STRENGTH FOR BEGINNERS

Exercise	Sets, Reps, Weight	Reference
Ball Squats	1–2 sets, 15 reps	Figure 6-21

Form Tips: Keep the abs in and the knees behind the toes as you squat. Add weights for more intensity.

Lunges	1–2 sets, 12 reps	Figure 6-23

Form Tips: Keep the front knee behind the toe as you lunge down.

▶ When creating a total-body routine, it's often hard to know which exercises you should include to get the most out of your exercise time. A general rule of thumb is to choose at least one exercise for each muscle group, adding more moves as you get stronger. For more ideas on total-body routines, visit my Total Body Workouts Index, which highlights workouts for all fitness levels. Visit http://about.com/exercise/totalbody.

Exercise	Sets, Reps, Weight	Reference
Leg Lifts on the Ball	1–2 sets, 12 reps	Figure 6-26

Form Tips: Keep the hips stacked and bend the bottom knee to support the body. Do this move on the floor for an easier modification.

Exercise	Sets, Reps, Weight	Reference
Inner Thigh Ball Squeeze	1–2 sets, 15 reps	Figure 6-28

Form Tips: Keep the abs contracted and keep tension on the ball throughout the exercise. For an easier modification, bend the knees and do the move from a seated position.

Exercise	Sets, Reps, Weight	Reference
Push-ups on the Ball	1–2 sets, 15 reps	Figure 6-5

Form Tips: For a variation, do the push-ups on the floor.

Exercise	Sets, Reps, Weight	Reference
Dumbbell Chest Press	1–2 sets, 15 reps, 5–10 pounds	Figure 6-1

Form Tips: Keep the abs in and bring the arms to only torso level when lowering the weights.

Exercise	Sets, Reps, Weight	Reference
Bent-Over Row	1–2 sets, 15 reps, 8–12 pounds	Figure 6-7

Form Tips: Keep the back flat and the elbow close to the body as you pull the weight up.

Exercise	Sets, Reps, Weight	Reference
Back Extension on the Ball	1–2 sets, 15 reps	Figure 6-12

Form Tips: Place the hands under the chin for an easier modification.

Exercise	Sets, Reps, Weight	Reference
Lateral Raise	1–2 sets, 12 reps, 3–8 pounds	Figure 6-14

Form Tips: Keep the elbows slightly bent and lift to only shoulder level.

Exercise	Sets, Reps, Weight	Reference
Biceps Curls	1–2 sets, 12 reps, 5–10 lbs	Figure 6-16

Form Tips: Use a slow and controlled movement rather than swinging the weights.

Exercise	Sets, Reps, Weight	Reference
Kickbacks	1–2 sets, 12 reps, 3–8 pounds	Figure 6-18

Form Tips: Keep the elbow in a fixed position as you straighten the arm.

Exercise	Sets, Reps, Weight	Reference
Ball Crunches	1–2 sets, 15 reps	Figure 6-32

Form Tips: Initiate the movement from the abs and try not to pull on the neck.

Exercise	Sets, Reps, Weight	Reference
Oblique Crunches on the Ball	1–2 sets, 15 reps on each side	Figure 6-33

Form Tips: Think of bringing the shoulder toward the opposite hip rather than bending the elbow toward the knee.

Exercise	Sets, Reps, Weight	Reference
Hamstring Stretch	1–2 reps, 10–30 seconds	Figure 7-1
Quad Stretch	1–2 reps, 10–30 seconds	Figure 7-2
Chest Stretch	1–2 reps, 10–30 seconds	Figure 7-5
Triceps Stretch	1–2 reps, 10–30 seconds	Figure 7-7

Total-Body Strength for the Beginner or Intermediate Level This workout is more challenging than the previous workout and includes new exercises, more sets, and, in some cases, increased weight. Adjust the exercises, weights, reps, and sets to fit your fitness level and goals. Before you get started, warm up with a few minutes of light cardio exercise.

TOTAL-BODY STRENGTH FOR BEGINNERS II

Exercise	Sets, Reps, Weight	Reference
Ball Squats	2 sets, 15 reps, 3–10 pounds	Figure 6-21

Form Tips: Walk the feet out enough that the knees stay behind the toes as you squat. Only go as low as you comfortably can.

Lunges	2 sets, 12 reps, 0–10 pounds	Figure 6-23

Form Tips: Keep the front knee behind the toe and push through the heel on the way up.

Crisscross Outer Thigh	2 sets, 15 reps, medium tube/band	Figure 6-27

Form Tips: Place the band over the feet and cross it in front, holding the ends in opposite hands. Keep the knees in alignment (don't let them turn in or out), and pull the band tighter to add more intensity.

Inner Thigh Ball Squeeze	2 sets, 15 reps	Figure 6-28

Form Tips: Keep the abs contracted and keep tension on the ball throughout the exercise.

Exercise	Sets, Reps, Weight	Reference
Push-ups on the Ball	2 sets, 12–15 reps	Figure 6-5

Form Tips: Contract the abs and keep the back straight throughout the movement.

Exercise	Sets, Reps, Weight	Reference
Chest Fly	2 sets, 15 reps, 5–8 pounds	Figure 6-2

Form Tips: Keep the elbows fixed and slightly bent and lower down to only torso level.

Exercise	Sets, Reps, Weight	Reference
Bent-Over Row	2 sets, 15 reps, 8 to 12 pounds	Figure 6-7

Form Tips: Keep the back flat and the elbow close to the body as you pull the weight up.

Exercise	Sets, Reps, Weight	Reference
Back Extension on the Ball	2 sets, 15 reps	Figure 6-12

Form Tips: Prop the feet against the wall if you need more stability.

Exercise	Sets, Reps, Weight	Reference
Overhead Press	2 sets, 15 reps, 5–8 pounds	Figure 6-13

Form Tips: Contract the abs to keep the back from arching as you push the weight overhead.

Exercise	Sets, Reps, Weight	Reference
Biceps Curls	2 sets, 15 reps, 5–10 pounds	Figure 6-16

Form Tips: Use a slow and controlled movement rather than swinging the weights.

Exercise	Sets, Reps, Weight	Reference
Triceps Kickbacks	2 sets, 15 reps, 3–8 pounds	Figure 6-18

Form Tips: Keep the elbow in a fixed position as you lift the weight.

Exercise	Sets, Reps, Weight	Reference
Modified Triceps Dips	2 sets, 12–15 reps	Figure 6-20

Form Tips: Keep the body close to the chair or bench as you lower down, and keep the shoulders away from the ears.

Exercise	Sets, Reps, Weight	Reference
Ball Crunches	2 sets, 15 reps	Figure 6-32

Form Tips: Initiate the movement from the abs and try not to pull on the neck.

Exercise	Sets, Reps, Weight	Reference
Oblique Crunches	2 sets, 15 reps on each side	Figure 6-33

Form Tips: Think of bringing the shoulder toward the opposite hip rather than bending the elbow toward the knee.

Exercise	Sets, Reps, Weight	Reference
Hamstring Stretch	1–2 reps, 10–30 seconds	Figure 7-1
Quad Stretch	1–2 reps, 10–30 seconds	Figure 7-2
Chest Stretch	1–2 reps, 10–30 seconds	Figure 7-5
Triceps Stretch	1–2 reps, 10–30 seconds	Figure 7-7

Total-Body Strength for Intermediate Exercisers This workout is more challenging than the previous workouts, with new exercises, more sets, and heavier weights. Adjust the workout to fit your fitness level and goals and make sure you warm up with light cardio or by doing warm-up sets of each exercise with light weight. Rest for 30 to 60 seconds (or more if needed) between sets.

TOTAL-BODY STRENGTH FOR INTERMEDIATE EXERCISERS

Exercise	Sets, Reps, Weights	Reference
Ball Squats	3 sets, 15 reps, 8–15 pounds	Figure 6-21

Form Tips: Walk the feet out enough that your knees stay behind the toes as you squat. Only go as low as you comfortably can.

Lunges	3 sets, 15 reps, 5–10 pounds	Figure 6-23

Form Tips: Keep the front knee behind the toe.

Crisscross Outer Thigh	3 sets, 15 reps, medium tube/band	Figure 6-27

Form Tips: Keep the knees in alignment and pull the band tighter to add more intensity.

Inner Thigh Ball Squeeze	3 sets, 15 reps	Figure 6-28

Form Tips: Keep the abs contracted and keep tension on the ball throughout the exercise.

Hamstring Rolls on the Ball	2 sets, 12 reps	Figure 6-29

Form Tips: Keep the hips lifted and the feet flexed throughout the exercise.

Exercise	Sets, Reps, Weights	Reference
Push-ups on the Ball	2 sets, 12–15 reps	Figure 6-5

Form Tips: Roll farther out on the ball for added intensity.

Exercise	Sets, Reps, Weights	Reference
Chest Fly	2 sets, 15 reps, 5–10 pounds	Figure 6-2

Keep the elbows fixed and slightly bent and lower down to only torso level.

Exercise	Sets, Reps, Weights	Reference
Dumbbell Chest Press	2 sets, 15 reps, 8–12 pounds	Figure 6-1

Form Tips: Keep the abs in and only lower the arms to torso level when lowering the weights.

Exercise	Sets, Reps, Weights	Reference
Bent-Over Row	2 sets, 15 reps, 10–15 pounds	Figure 6-7

Form Tips: Keep the back flat and the elbow close to the body as you pull the weight up.

Exercise	Sets, Reps, Weights	Reference
Overhead Press	2 sets, 15 reps, 5–8 pounds	Figure 6-13

Form Tips: Contract the abs to keep the back from arching as you push the weight overhead.

Exercise	Sets, Reps, Weights	Reference
Lateral Raise	2 sets, 12 reps, 5–10 pounds	Figure 6-14

Form Tips: Keep the elbows slightly bent and lift to only shoulder level.

Exercise	Sets, Reps, Weights	Reference
Biceps Curls	2 sets, 15 reps, 5–10 pounds	Figure 6-16

Form Tips: Turn the palms in to incorporate more of the forearms.

Exercise	Sets, Reps, Weights	Reference
Lying Triceps Extensions	2 sets, 15 reps, 3–8 pounds	Figure 6-19

Form Tips: Lower the weights until elbows are at 90 degrees.

Exercise	Sets, Reps, Weights	Reference
Triceps Dips	2 sets, 15 reps	Figure 6-20

Form Tips: Keep the body close to the chair or bench as you lower down, and keep the shoulders away from the ears.

Exercise	Sets, Reps, Weights	Reference
Oblique Crunches	2 sets, 15 reps on each side	Figure 6-33

Form Tips: Think of bringing the shoulder toward the opposite hip rather than bending the elbow toward the knee.

Exercise	Sets, Reps, Weights	Reference
Ball Crunches	2 sets, 15 reps	Figure 6-32

Form Tips: Pull the abs in tight to bring the body into a C shape as you crunch up.

Exercise	Sets, Reps, Weights	Reference
Bicycles	2 sets, 16 reps on each side	Figure 6-36

Form Tips: Bring your knees in toward the chest and slowly go through a pedaling motion, touching the left elbow to the right knee, then the right elbow to the left knee.

Exercise	Sets, Reps, Weights	Reference
Hamstring Stretch	1–2 reps, 10–30 seconds	Figure 7-1
Quad Stretch	1–2 reps, 10–30 seconds	Figure 7-2
Calf Stretch	1–2 reps, 10–30 seconds	Figure 7-3
Chest Stretch	1–2 reps, 10–30 seconds	Figure 7-5
Triceps Stretch	1–2 reps, 10–30 seconds	Figure 7-7

Targeted Workouts

Once you've mastered total-body workouts and are ready to progress, one option is to try a split routine. The most common split involves doing an upper-body workout and a lower-body workout on alternating or separate days. By splitting your routine, you'll not only be adding more exercises, you'll also be adding more strength-training days to your routine. Like the total-body routines, you want to work your muscles at least two times a week, so if you're following an upper body/lower body split, that means you'll be lifting weights about four times a week.

Upper Body this upper-body workout involves a variety of exercises targeting the chest, back, shoulders, and arms. For each exercise, you'll be doing 2 to 3 sets, depending on your goals and fitness level. Choose a weight that will allow you to do 12 reps of each exercise with good form … the last rep should be difficult but not impossible. Rest about 30 to 60 seconds between sets, and adjust any aspect of the workout so that you're challenged but not in pain. Before you get started, warm up with a few minutes of light cardio or perform a warm-up set of each exercise with light weights.

UPPER BODY

Exercise	Sets, Reps, Weights	Reference
Ball Push-ups	2–3 sets, 12 reps	Figure 6-5

Form Tips: To make the move easier, position the ball under the knees/shins. To make it harder, roll out until the ball is under the ankles or toes.

Exercise	Sets, Reps, Weights	Reference
Incline Chest Press	2–3 sets, 12 reps, 8–15 pounds	Figure 6-1

Form Tips: Keep the incline at about a 45-degree angle to avoid straining the shoulders.

Exercise	Sets, Reps, Weights	Reference
Chest Fly	2–3 sets, 12 reps, 8–12 pounds	Figure 6-2

Form Tips: Do this on a ball for more intensity.

Exercise	Sets, Reps, Weights	Reference
Bent-Over Row	2–3 sets, 12 reps, 12–20 pounds	Figure 6-7

Form Tips: Keep the back flat and the elbows close to the body as you pull the weight up.

Exercise	Sets, Reps, Weights	Reference
Dumbbell Pullover	2–3 sets, 12 reps, 10–15 pounds	Figure 6-9

Form Tips: Keep the elbows slightly bent and lower the arms to only about ear level.

Exercise	Sets, Reps, Weights	Reference
Bent-Over Reverse Fly	2 sets, 12 reps, 5–10 pounds	Figure 6-11

Form Tips: Contract the abs to support the back and lift the arms to only shoulder level.

Exercise	Sets, Reps, Weights	Reference
Overhead Press	2 sets, 12 reps, 8–12 pounds	Figure 6-13

Form Tips: Make the move more difficult by standing up or even standing on one leg

Exercise	Sets, Reps, Weights	Reference
Front Raise	2 sets, 12 reps, 5–10 pounds	Figure 6-15

Form Tips: Lift the arms to shoulder level and keep the elbows slightly bent to protect the joints.

Exercise	Sets, Reps, Weights	Reference
Lateral Raise	2 sets, 12 reps, 5–10 pounds	Figure 6-14

Form Tips: Keep the elbows slightly bent and lift to only shoulder level.

Exercise	Sets, Reps, Weights	Reference
Biceps Curls	2 sets, 12 reps, 8–12 pounds	Figure 6-16

Form Tips: Vary the move by trying this with a barbell or cables.

Exercise	Sets, Reps, Weights	Reference
Concentration Curls	2 sets, 12 reps, 8–12 pounds	Figure 6-17

Form Tips: Prop the elbow on the inside of the thigh for leverage and curl the weight toward the shoulder.

Exercise	Sets, Reps, Weights	Reference
Triceps Dips	2 sets, 12 reps	Figure 6-20

Form Tips: Make the move harder by walking the feet out.

Exercise	Sets, Reps, Weights	Reference
Lying Triceps Extensions	2 sets, 10–12 reps, 5–10 pounds	Figure 6-19

Form Tips: Lower the weights until elbows are at 90 degrees.

Exercise	Sets, Reps, Weights	Reference
Chest Stretch	1–2 reps, 10–30 seconds	Figure 7-5
Triceps Stretch	1–2 reps, 10–30 seconds	Figure 7-7
Shoulder Stretch	1–2 reps, 10–30 seconds	Figure 7-6

TOOLS YOU NEED

When splitting your workouts, you don't have to follow an upper body/lower body split. Just keep in mind that you don't want to work the same muscle groups two days in a row. Many exercisers find that separating upper- and lower-body exercises makes it easy to keep track of workouts and exercises. For some ideas on different types of upper-body workouts you can try, visit my Upper Body Workouts Index at http://about.com/exercise/upperbody.

ASK YOUR GUIDE

How often should I work my abs for maximum results?

One popular myth about the abs is that you should train them every day to get them flat. First, ab exercises won't reduce the fat over the abs—that can happen only by losing body fat. Second, your abs require rest just like the rest of your body. The key is to make sure you choose a variety of exercises to challenge each part of the abs.

Lower Body The following workout includes more advanced lower-body exercises targeting the quads, glutes, hips, hamstrings, and calves. Warm up with light cardio or a warm-up set of each exercise with light weights.

LOWER BODY

Exercise	Sets, Reps, Weights	Reference
Barbell Squats	2–3 sets, 12 reps, 10–50 pounds	Figure 6-21

Form Tips: Use a spotter if you're lifting very heavy. Modify this exercise by switching to dumbbells or doing a leg press.

One-Legged Squats	2–3 sets, 12 reps	Figure 6-22

Form Tips: Use caution when trying this exercise and avoid squatting too low. Modify this move by doing it without the ball and holding onto a wall or chair for balance.

Deadlifts	2–3 sets, 12 reps, 10–15 pounds	Figure 6-24

Form Tips: Keep the shoulders back and the back flat throughout the movement.

One-Legged Deadlifts	2–3 sets, 12 reps, 8–12 pounds	Figure 6-25

Form Tips: Form Tips: Lightly touch the back foot to the floor for balance and keep the back flat as you lower down.

Lunges	2 sets, 12 reps, 5–10 pounds	Figure 6-23

Form Tips: Step forward with the right leg and lower into a lunge. Push off the left foot and lunge forward, alternating sides.

Exercise	Sets, Reps	Reference
Lunges	2 sets, 12 reps, 8–12 pounds	Figure 6-23

Form Tips: Hold one dumbbell in front of the chest and lunge from side to side. Sit back on the heels to target the glutes and keep the knees behind the toes.

Exercise	Sets, Reps	Reference
Leg Lifts on the Ball	2 sets, 16 reps	Figure 6-26

Form Tips: Keep the hips stacked and bend the bottom knee to support the body. Do this move on the floor for an easier modification.

Exercise	Sets, Reps	Reference
Inner Thigh Ball Squeeze	2 sets, 16 reps	Figure 6-28

Form Tips: Keep the abs contracted and keep tension on the ball throughout the exercise.

Exercise	Sets, Reps	Reference
Hamstring Rolls on the Ball	2 sets, 16 reps	Figure 6-29

Form Tips: Keep the hips lifted and the feet flexed throughout the exercise.

Exercise	Sets, Reps	Reference
Calf Raises	2 sets, 16 reps	Figure 6-31

Form Tips: Stand on a step or bench to get full range of motion.

Exercise	Sets, Reps	Reference
Hamstring Stretch	1–2 reps, 10–30 seconds	Figure 7-1
Quad Stretch	1–2 reps, 10–30 seconds	Figure 7-2
Calf Stretch	1–2 reps, 10–30 seconds	Figure 7-3
Hip Stretch	1–2 reps, 10–30 seconds	Figure 7-4

Core Workout When splitting up your workouts, you can either work your core on separate days from your other strength-training workouts or add a core workout at the end if you have the time. You should treat your abs just like any other muscle and give them at least one day of rest before working them again.

The following workout includes a variety of moves, some of which require an exercise ball. Many of these exercises can be challenging, so use caution and take the time to practice the moves with good form and balance.

CORE WORKOUT

Exercise	Sets, Reps	Reference
Crunches on the Ball	3 sets, 15 reps	Figure 6-32

Form Tips: Pull the abs in tight to bring the body into a C shape as you crunch up.

Oblique Crunches on the Ball	3 sets, 15 reps on each side	Figure 6-33

Form Tips: Keep the ball stable as you crunch up and to the side.

Reverse Crunches	3 sets, 15 reps	Figure 6-35

Form Tips: Initiate the movement from the abs and lift the hips off the floor without swinging the legs.

Knee Tucks on the Ball	2 sets, 10–15 reps	Figure 6-34

Form Tips: Position the ball under the shins and contract the abs as you pull the knees in.

Exercise	Sets, Reps	Reference
Bicycle	2 sets, 8 reps on each side	Figure 6-36

Form Tips: Try to keep the belly as flat as you can throughout the movement.

Exercise	Sets, Reps	Reference
Back Extension on the Ball	2 sets, 15 reps	Figure 6-12

Form Tips: Prop the feet against the wall if you need more stability.

Workouts for Travelers

Traveling can make it tough to fit in exercise. You're out of your element and away from your usual schedule and workout equipment, which makes it easy to blow off exercise altogether. You may find it easier to get some exercise in if you engage in workouts that are short, easy to follow, and can be done with little or no equipment. You may not be doing the same workouts you do at home, but you can maintain your strength and endurance so that getting back to your workouts will be a piece of cake.

The following workouts offer some ideas for how you can squeeze in short workouts while on the road. These workouts don't follow traditional strength guidelines and often have you doing exercise for a certain length of time rather than standard sets or reps. They're also circuit-type workouts, which have you going from one exercise to another with little or no rest. While this type of workout won't help you gain a lot of strength or size, it's great for maintaining strength and endurance while you're on the road.

No-Equipment Travel Workout The following workout includes a variety of exercises that can be done with nothing more than a chair (or bed) and your own body weight. To do this workout, complete each exercise for the suggested duration (or modify according to your fitness level) and move on to the next exercise after a brief rest. Complete the circuit once for a 10-minute workout or go through it again for a longer workout.

NO-EQUIPMENT TRAVEL WORKOUT

Exercise	Duration	Reference
Ball Squats	1 minute	Figure 6-21

Form Tips: Squat to a chair if you don't have a ball and add weights for more intensity.

Exercise	Duration	Reference
Lunges	1 minute	Figure 6-23

Form Tips: 30 seconds on each side.

Exercise	Duration	Reference
Lunges	1 minute	Figure 6-23

Form Tips: Sit back in the heels to target the glutes and keep the knees behind the toes.

Exercise	Duration	Reference
Leg Extensions	1 minute	Figure 6-30

Form Tips: Sit with abs in and spine straight as you straighten one leg up and down for 30 seconds. Repeat on the other leg.

Exercise	Duration	Reference
Bent-Over Reverse Fly, No Weights	1 minute	Figure 6-11

Form Tips: Turn the thumbs up to the ceiling and lift the arms to shoulder level, contracting the upper back muscles.

Exercise	Duration	Reference
Push-ups on the Ball	1 minute	Figure 6-5

Form Tips: Do this move on the knees or toes. If you need to, rest after 30 seconds and then complete the minute.

Triceps Dips	1 minute	Figure 6-20

Form Tips: Keep the body close to the chair or bench as you lower down and keep the shoulders away from the ears. Rest halfway through if needed.

Crunches on the Ball	1 minute	Figure 6-32

Form Tips: Do this move on the floor if you don't have a ball.

Oblique Crunches	1 minute	Figure 6-33

Form Tips: Do this move on the floor if you don't have a ball.

Back Extension on the Ball	1 minute	Figure 6-12

Form Tips: Do this move on the floor if you don't have a ball.

Travel Workout with Resistance Tubes Resistance bands or tubes make great travel companions; they don't take up much room and you can use them for a variety of resistance-training exercises. The following workout includes exercises you can do using resistance tubes while traveling. This workout follows a circuit format where you move from one exercise to the next with little or no rest. Adjust the workout as needed to fit your fitness level.

Exercise	Duration	Reference
Chest Press with Resistance Tube	1 minute	Figure 6-3

Form Tips: Wrap the tube around a sturdy object behind you and move forward to create tension as you press the arms out and in, contracting the chest.

Exercise	Duration	Reference
Push-ups with Resistance Tube	30 seconds–1 minute	Figure 6-6

Form Tips: Wrap the tube around your back and grab each side in your hands to add intensity to regular push-ups.

Exercise	Duration	Reference
Bent-Over Row with Resistance Tube	1 minute	Figure 6-8

Form Tips: Place the tube under the feet and hold onto both sides as you pull the elbows up toward the torso, squeezing the back.

Exercise	Duration	Reference
Seated Row with Resistance Tube	1 minute	Figure 6-10

Form Tips: Wrap the tube around a sturdy object and hold handles in both hands, arms straight out in front. Bend the elbows to pull the arms into a row, arms parallel to the floor.

Exercise	Duration	Reference
Overhead Press	1 minute	Figure 6-13

Form Tips: Place tube under feet (standing or sitting) and hold handles in both hands to press the weight overhead.

Exercise	Duration	Reference
Biceps Curls with Resistance Tube	1 minute	Figure 6-16

Form Tips: Place tube under feet and hold handles in both hands. Bend the elbows and curl the hands toward the shoulders.

Triceps Dips	1 minute	Figure 6-20

Form Tips: Keep the body close to the chair or bench as you lower down and keep the shoulders away from the ears. Rest halfway through if needed.

Ball Squats	1 minute	Figure 6-21

Form Tips: Keep the abs in and the knees behind the toes as you squat.

Lunges	1 minute	Figure 6-23

Form Tips: 30 seconds on each side.

Lunges	1 minute	Figure 6-23

Form Tips: Sit back in the heels to target the glutes and keep the knees behind the toes.

ELSEWHERE ON THE WEB

▶ Nothing gets a busy exerciser's attention more than the phrase *time-saver workout*. The good news is that there are plenty of resources out there for people who want shorter, quality workouts. Many gyms now offer express workouts that can be done in less than thirty minutes, and if you're a video fan, there are a number of choices for time-saving home workouts. One of my favorites is Cathe Friedrich's Timesaver Series, available at www.cathe.com.

Timesaver Workout

Fitting in exercise is easy when you have the time, but what if you don't? If you're like most people, you probably skip your workout altogether. But there are creative ways to squeeze in strength-training workouts if you don't have a lot of time. One way to save time is to combine upper- and lower-body moves so you're working more than one muscle at the same time, such as a squat with an overhead press. You can also choose compound exercises (like push-ups, lunges, and triceps dips) to make sure you're working more muscles at a time.

The following workout offers both compound movements and combination exercises set out in a circuit format where you move from one exercise to another with little or no rest. When combining exercises, take your time and start with lighter weights since the exercises may be more challenging. Complete one circuit for a 10-minute workout or repeat the circuit one or more times for a longer workout.

10-MINUTE TOTAL BODY TIMESAVER

Exercise	Duration, Weights
Squats with Overhead Press	1 minute, 5–10 pounds

Form Tips: Hold the weights above the shoulders as you squat and press them overhead as you stand.

Ball Push-ups	1 minute

Form Tips: To make the move easier, position the ball under the knees/shins. To make it harder, roll out until the ball is under the ankles or toes.

Exercise	Duration, Weights
Lunge with Lateral Raise	1 minute, 3–8 pounds

Form Tips: Lift the arms out to the sides as you lower into a lunge. Do 30 seconds on each leg.

Push-ups with Resistance Bands	1 minute

Form Tips: Wrap a band or tube around your back and hold in each hand to add intensity during push-ups.

Deadlifts with Bent-Over Row	1 minute, 8–15 pounds

Form Tips: Lower into a deadlift with weights in front of you and pull the weights in, squeezing the back. Lower the arms and return to start.

Hamstring Roll with Leg Lift	30 seconds–1 minute

Form Tips: With heels on the ball, lift the hips and squeeze the hamstrings to roll the ball in. Roll back out and lift the right leg off the ball, holding for 1–2 seconds. Lower and roll the ball in again, repeating the leg lift with the left leg.

Ball Push-ups with Knee Tucks	1 minute

Form Tips: In push-up position with ball under the legs, lower into a push-up. Push back up and tuck the knees, rolling the ball in and squeezing the abs. Roll the ball back and repeat, alternating push-ups and knee tucks.

TOOLS YOU NEED

▸ When you have unexpected interruptions in your usual routine, you may think doing shorter workouts is a waste of time. But short workouts can be just as effective if you do the right exercises. Saving time is about being creative, but it's hard to know how to get the most out of your workout time. My article "10-Minute Timesaver Workouts" offers tips for creating short, effective cardio and strength-training workouts to fit your busy schedule. Visit http://about.com/exercise/10minuteworkouts.

Exercise	Duration, Weights
Modified Triceps Dips	1 minute

Form Tips: Keep the body close to the chair or bench as you lower down, and keep the shoulders away from the ears.

Lunges with Biceps Curls	30 seconds on each side, 5–10 pounds

Form Tips: Curl the weights up as you lower into a lunge.

Crunches	1 minute

Form Tips: Perform each crunch by lifting up for 2 counts and down for 2 counts.

Get Linked

The following resources at my **About.com** *Exercise site offer a variety of workout ideas for beginner, intermediate, and advanced exercisers.*

BEGINNER EXERCISER

If you've never exercised or it's been awhile since you picked up a dumbbell, start with these beginner workouts. They require very little equipment and provide a strong foundation for your body.

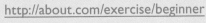 http://about.com/exercise/beginner

INTERMEDIATE EXERCISER

If you've been exercising for several weeks and have some basic knowledge of strength training and cardio exercise, these intermediate workouts will give you some ideas for how to challenge yourself with new and interesting exercises.

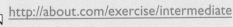 http://about.com/exercise/intermediate

ADVANCED EXERCISER

If you've been exercising regularly for more than three months, you may be bored with the usual workouts. These advanced workouts offer great variety for the exerciser who's ready to try something new.

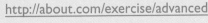 http://about.com/exercise/advanced

Chapter 8. Workouts to Suit Your Schedule and Goals | 155

The **ABOUT**.com *Guide to* **Getting in Shape**

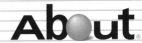

Chapter 9

Setting Up a Complete Program

Tips for Scheduling and Sticking with Workouts

Looking at all the different elements of a fitness program, it may seem impossible to fit it all in. There's cardio, strength training, yoga, Pilates, and stretching, each requiring its own equipment, time, and focus. It is possible to fit it all in, but if you're a beginner, you don't necessarily have to. It's always best to start with a simple program that fits with your schedule and needs rather than try to cram every activity in at once. Anytime you start exercising, you may be doing activities that are new to you and require some time to build skills, experience, and conditioning. It's often best to keep the new activities to a minimum to avoid confusion and give yourself time to perfect each type of exercise.

When scheduling your workouts, there are a few basic rules that will help you figure out where to start:

If I do cardio and strength in the same workout, which one should I do first?

When setting up your workout, go by your goals. If you want to get strong, do strength training first so you can give it your all. If you want to build endurance, go for cardio before strength training. If you want to lose weight and get fit, try different combinations to find what feels good to you.

- **Cardio workouts can usually be done every day.** If you do very intense workouts or you're just getting started, you may need to rest the day after, but most moderate workouts can be done on consecutive days.
- **Cardio and strength training can be done together or separately.** It's always best to keep cardio and strength training separate so you can give each your full energy and attention. But it's fine to do them both in the same workout or on the same day if you have a busy schedule.
- **Workouts can be broken up throughout the day.** As mentioned previously, you don't need large chunks of time for exercise. It's possible to get a good workout by splitting it into several shorter workouts throughout the day.
- **You can exercise at any time of day.** Make sure you choose a time that's right for you and isn't too close to bedtime, since that can interrupt your sleep.

Scheduling workouts is a piece of cake, though sticking with them is usually the tricky part. It helps to put your weight-loss goals aside for the first few weeks to focus all your energy and attention on showing up for your workouts. That helps take the pressure off so you can focus on more tangible, practical steps to reach your goal. What that means is making it as easy as possible for you to keep your commitment to exercise. Think for a moment about the obstacles that often get in the way of your workouts. You may feel tired or hungry, or perhaps you forgot to pack your gym bag the night before. Showing up for your workouts means getting rid of all the obstacles before they happen.

Some ideas include:

- **Pack your bag.** If you're going to the gym, pack your bag the night before and put it by the door. If you pack it in the morning, you're more likely to be rushed and forget something or get frustrated and forget it altogether.

- **Get your clothes ready.** If you're working out at home or outside in the morning, put your workout clothes and shoes next to the bed. As soon as you get up, get dressed before you do anything else.
- **Plan your meals and snacks.** It's not much fun (or terribly productive) to work out when you're starving. Get your meals and snacks ready so that you always have fuel available before and after exercise.
- **Be flexible.** If you're tired after a long day at work, don't skip your workout, but instead, decide on a shorter, more moderate workout or allow yourself some extra time to warm up, stretch, or sit in the hot tub.
- **Say no.** If people make demands on your time and you tend to cave, treat your workout time like it's an important business meeting or other appointment you'd never miss … there's nothing more important than your health and well-being.

Creating a Workout Schedule

When scheduling workouts, you may have to experiment to find the right fit for your schedule and lifestyle. What works one week may not work the next, so your best friend will often be your ability to be flexible. You may find you need to change how you do things to fit in exercise, getting help with the kids so you can exercise in the morning or bringing your own food to work so you can exercise during your lunch hour. The key is to be willing to shuffle things around to fit in exercise, remembering that taking the time to work out can give you more energy so you can get more things done.

With those ideas in mind, the following steps will help you map out your workout schedule and set some goals for yourself. Be honest and realistic when planning out your workout time. Remember,

TOOLS YOU NEED

There are any number of reasons we don't exercise, from busy schedules to that naughty little voice inside that finds all kinds of excuses to skip the workout. Part of being consistent with exercise is figuring out what's standing in your way and, more importantly, how to get rid of those obstacles and excuses. For specific ways to deal with this, check out my article "Why You Don't Exercise," at http://about .com/exercise/whyno exercise.

your goals should be attainable, so choose a schedule you know you can follow with 100 percent commitment.

1. Get out your day planner or calendar and choose how many days you'll exercise.
2. Determine how much time you have available to spend on your workouts.
3. Decide what type of cardio and strength-training exercises you'll do.
4. Commit to following your exercise plan for one month to see how it works with your schedule and goals. If something isn't working, you can reevaluate your plan and make any changes you may need.
5. Decide how you'll reward yourself for sticking to your plan each week.

To see this step-by-step plan in action, imagine you've decided to exercise four days a week for about forty-five minutes at a time using some of the cardio and strength workouts presented here. You might plan a workout schedule that looks something like this:

Day 1	Beginner Interval Workout (20 minutes), Yoga Exercises (10–20 minutes)
Day 2	Total Body Strength for Beginners (about 20–30 minutes)
Day 3	Rest
Day 4	Moderate Cardio Workout (30 Minutes), Stretching Exercises
Day 5	Rest
Day 6	Beginner Interval Workout, Total Body Strength for Beginners
Day 7	Rest

Being consistent with exercise is all about being committed, disciplined, and motivated. But being so responsible all the time is tough unless you have something fun to look forward to. Rewarding yourself for your exercise accomplishments is one way to stay motivated. When you know there's something good waiting for you at the end of the week, you'll be more likely to stick with the program. Try a massage, a new CD, or a weekend getaway.

Another way to look at your workout schedule is to figure out how many workouts you want to complete for the week and then fit them into your schedule. For example, say you want to start a beginner program with three cardio workouts, two strength-training workouts, and one Pilates workout. You could plan to do cardio on Monday, Wednesday, and Friday; strength training on Tuesday and Thursday; and Pilates on the weekend. If working out every day seems like too much at once, you could combine some of your cardio and strength workouts. Just make sure you work out for a reasonable amount of time and don't wear yourself out too much.

Have a Backup Plan

Sticking with your workouts is all about having a plan and being prepared. But as you probably know, even the best-laid plans can turn to dust in the face of life's little interruptions. There will be days when everything goes your way and you fit in your workout with no problems. Then there are the other days, the ones where you wake up late, a child gets sick, you forget your running shoes, or you end up working late because of your crazy boss. Obviously there are times when other things should take priority over your workouts. But having a backup plan and being ready for unexpected schedule changes can help you keep the momentum you need to stick with your program.

- Keep an extra gym bag in your desk at work with some basics: a pair of athletic shoes, some resistance bands, a towel, etc. If you have to work late unexpectedly, use your lunch hour for a quick walk or run or do some exercises with your resistance bands whenever you find a few extra minutes.

▶ For those long days at the office or on the road, you might consider something a little different. Yourself!Fitness is an interactive exercise program that works on your PC or Xbox. Maya, your virtual personal trainer, can create a workout plan that fits your schedule and whatever equipment you have available. This is a great option for exercising in your hotel. Check out my review at http://about.com/exercise/yourselffitness to learn more.

- Keep an extra pair of athletic shoes in the car; if you can't make it to the gym, stop on the way home from work at a park or track and go for a quick walk.

- Make a list of workout ideas; if you can't do your usual cardio or strength-training workout, what could you do instead? Make a list of everything you can think of (run up and down the stairs at work for five to ten minutes, do a minute of squats in between phone calls, etc.) and keep it handy. The next time you have to miss your workout, get out your list and see how many things you can check off.

- Have some home workouts to try; you may prefer to work out at the gym, but sometimes it's just more convenient to exercise at home. Keep some workout videos or a few sets of weights around so you can at least get some type of activity in.

Sample Schedules

There are a number of ways to set up a workout schedule, but the key is to make sure you fit in all the elements of a balanced program (cardio, strength, and flexibility) in whatever way works for you. Below are some suggestions for different workout options, whether you want to exercise three days a week or six days a week. Experts recommend working out for no more than an hour at a time since longer workouts typically have higher drop-out rates, so keep that in mind when mapping out your plan.

The sample schedules below are just a starting point for you to set up your own plan.

Day I	Cardio (20–30 minutes)/Total Body Strength (20 minutes)
Day 2	Rest
Day 3	Cardio (30 or more minutes)/Yoga or Pilates
Day 4	Rest
Day 5	Cardio (20–30 minutes)/Total Body Strength (20 minutes)
Day 6	Rest
Day 7	Rest

OPTION 2: 4 DAYS PER WEEK

Day I	Cardio (20–45 minutes)
Day 2	Total Body Strength/Stretching
Day 3	Rest
Day 4	Cardio (20–30 minutes)/Yoga or Pilates
Day 5	Cardio (20–45 minutes)
Day 6	Rest
Day 7	Rest

OPTION 3: 5 DAYS PER WEEK

Day I	Cardio (20–30 minutes)/ Upper Body
Day 2	Cardio (20–30 minutes)/Yoga or Pilates
Day 3	Lower Body Strength/Stretching
Day 4	Rest
Day 5	Cardio (20–30 minutes)/Stretching
Day 6	Total Body Strength
Day 7	Rest

Day 1	Cardio and Chest/Shoulders/Triceps
Day 2	Lower Body/Stretching
Day 3	Cardio (20–45 minutes)
Day 4	Cardio and Back/Biceps
Day 5	Rest
Day 6	Cardio (20–45 minutes)
Day 7	Yoga or Pilates

It's best to have at least one rest day each week (or more, if you're a beginner), although it's fine to try to do something active every day. Save your light walking or gentle stretching routines for your rest days so you're still active but your body has a chance to rest from the more intense workouts.

Make Your Workouts Fun

People don't often put the words *fun* and *exercise* in the same sentence. Having fun is when you get to go to the beach or throw a barbecue in the backyard. Exercise is more like, well, exercise. Not every workout is going to be fun, but there are some ways to make your workouts more appealing.

Music is one of the best ways to make exercise more fun and energetic. There's nothing like hearing your favorite song just when you're ready to give up, and these days, there are a number of options for listening to music while you exercise. The most popular are MP3 players, on which you can download your favorite music and make your own exercise playlists. The nice thing about MP3 players is that you can often download a variety of things to listen to, including audiobooks, podcasts, and even workouts. Some music software like iTunes will also have playlists created by other listeners, so you can often find great ideas for music to help you move.

Another way to make workouts more fun is to exercise with a friend or family member. Having a regular appointment to get together for a walk or gym workout with someone else makes it harder for you to skip your workout. Not only that, but your workout will go by much faster when you have someone to talk to. Group fitness is another good motivator; there's an energy you get when working out with other people that you may not feel when exercising alone. You can choose a gym class or an outdoor walking or running club, and there are even walking clubs out there for parents who want to exercise with their kids.

One expanding area of fitness is outdoor boot-camp-style workouts, where an instructor takes you through a variety of exercises and activities to push you a little harder. Look in your local paper or phone book to see what's offered in your area.

Another option for making exercise more fun is to play some games. There are a number of great board games and computer games out there designed to get you moving while having fun. Some of the latest computer games include Dance Dance Revolution, a PlayStation game that has you following dance steps on the screen. EyeToy: Kinetic, which also works with PlayStation, is an innovative game that offers virtual personal training with a variety of workouts, from cardio and combat to mind/body and toning. There are also board games you can play with your family, like The Fitness Challenge, available at many bookstores and discount stores, which challenges you and a partner to exercise for eight weeks with incentives and rewards to stay on track.

When searching for ways to make workouts more fun, the best role model you can find is a child. With kids, anything can become a game—playing tag, chasing each other around the yard, or tossing a football. Playing with your kids is a great way to remember

▶ Motivation comes in all shapes and sizes, and if you have a computer, you can often find exercise motivation and support right on the Internet. One hot Web site is PEERtrainer, which allows you to join or create a fitness group with people who have goals similar to yours. You can log workouts, meals, and goals and use your group members for support and encouragement. Visit www .peertrainer.com.

what it was like to be young and carefree, just moving around with no other agenda than having some fun and whiling away the hours. Try playing some kids' games like hopscotch or tag or take the kids to the park once a week to chase butterflies or toss a baseball. Find ways to recapture the joy of moving and you may find you start to enjoy exercise.

Get Linked

The following resources at my **About.com** *Exercise site offer you more ideas for planning your exercise strategy, setting up a program, and finding ways to make exercise more enjoyable.*

HOW TO EXERCISE AND LOSE WEIGHT ON A BUSY SCHEDULE

Finding time to exercise can be tough unless you take some time to plan how you'll make exercise a priority. This article offers specific tips for fitting in exercise even when you're busy.

 http://about.com/exercise/busyschedule

EXERCISE FORUM

The Exercise Forum is a great place to come when you have questions or need support for sticking with your exercise program. It's free to join and you'll find plenty of topics to discuss.

 http://exercise.about.com/mpboards.htm

FITTING IN EXERCISE

This article breaks down each element of a complete exercise program (cardio, strength training, and flexibility) and explains how much and how often you should do each one. It also includes a checklist for making sure you fit everything in.

http://about.com/exercise/fittinginexercise

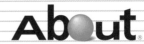

Chapter 10

Nutrition and Getting in Shape

Keeping a Food Journal

Back in the first part of this book, we talked about setting weight-loss goals, and part of that process involved determining your BMR (basal metabolic rate) to learn how many calories your body needs to function as well as determining how many calories you burn with exercise and activity. This is important for losing weight since diet is the most important component of your weight-loss program. Keeping track of what you're eating on a daily basis may be a necessary step if you want to lose weight.

Studies have found that people who keep food journals to track their eating during the week are more likely to lose weight. It's not just about counting calories, but about being aware of when you eat and why you eat. We all know we should eat only when we're hungry, but most of us have reached for that bag of chips or box

▶ Emotional eating is something most of us do from time to time, but if you do it too often, you can sabotage your efforts to get in shape and lose weight. Food can be a comfort when you're stressed, depressed, bored, or lonely, giving a temporary boost to your mood. Learn new ways of dealing with your emotions in my article "Are You an Emotional Eater?" at http://about.com/ exercise/emotionaleater.

of cookies because we're bored, depressed, or lonely. Keeping a food journal can give you insight into habits you may not even be aware of.

For example, I had a client who swore she was eating healthy but couldn't manage to lose weight. After keeping a food journal for a week, she noticed she was eating almost twenty Hershey's Kisses a day, which added up to almost 500 extra daily calories. Before she kept the journal, she would walk by the front desk at work and pick up a few throughout the day, thinking a few here and there wouldn't matter. But when she counted them, she was shocked at how many she was actually eating.

There are different ways to keep a food journal, some more complicated than others. The simplest way is to get a notebook, write the date at the top of the page, and list everything you eat each day. To get an accurate count of your calories, you'll need to measure whenever you can, read food labels to get serving size and calorie information, and perhaps use an online food database for meals eaten out.

You can also use books such as *The Pocket Food & Exercise Diary* by Allan Borushek or *DietMinder Personal Food & Fitness Journal* by Frances E. Wilkins, both of which can be found at major bookstores or ordered online. These journals often have detailed forms where you can track your food and exercise as well as information on portion sizes, basic nutrition, and the nutritional content of common foods. However you decide to track your eating, the basic elements to track include:

- What time you eat
- The calories of each meal and total calories for the day
- Fat grams
- Amount of carbs

- Amount of protein
- Fiber intake
- Water and/or fluid intake
- Any vitamins or other supplements you're taking

You can also keep track of your serving sizes to help reduce your calories. This is especially important since food portions have grown tremendously over the last twenty years, even though the recommended servings haven't. Just visit any bagel shop and you'll find that bagels have grown to roughly the size of your head. A reasonable serving is actually the size of a hockey puck.

Keep in mind that a portion size isn't the same thing as a serving size. A serving is the amount of food recommended by the USDA in the food-guide pyramid, whereas a portion describes the amount of food you actually eat. In other words, you can get a portion of spaghetti at a restaurant and it might contain more than three servings.

The whole portion-size thing can be confusing, but there are some ways to visualize the correct portion of food with some simple comparisons:

- 3 ounces of meat or fish = a deck of cards or the palm of your hand (no fingers!)
- 1 ounce of cheese = four dice
- 1 cup of pasta = a tennis ball
- 1 serving of veggies or fruit = about the size of a fist
- 1 serving of peanut butter = a golf ball

There are some simple ways to cut your portions and save calories without tracking a thing. If you eat out and your portions are huge, have the waiter put half in a doggie bag or share an entrée. Using smaller plates and bowls can also help you control your

ELSEWHERE ON THE WEB

▶ The Food Diary, offered by About.com's Weight Loss Guide, is a great way to keep track of what you eat and drink for each meal, what time you usually eat, and how many times you snack each day. The diary also includes a section for emotional eating, which can help you pinpoint those times you eat when you're not hungry. By recording your feelings, you can find new ways to deal with your emotions. Visit http://about.com/weightloss/fooddiary.

portions—the bigger the plate, the more you'll want to fill it. Being mindful of how much you're eating and knowing you'll be writing it down will be a big help in controlling your eating.

Another way to track your calories is by using an online tracking service that includes a food database such as FitWatch.com or FitDay.com. These food databases make it easy to track not only your calories but also the nutrients you're getting. For example, if you use the food database at FitWatch, each item you choose will come up with a label that contains the same information you'd find on a typical food label, including calories, water, carbs, protein, fat, cholesterol, and fiber, just to name a few. By using an online service, you can log on at any time throughout the day and enter information for each meal and snack. CalorieKing.com is another great resource, offering food databases for a number of popular fast-food restaurants. And don't forget, many restaurants now post nutritional information on their Web sites so you can do a little research before you head out for dinner.

Eating Healthy Calories

As mentioned before, losing weight is all about burning more calories than you eat. By that definition, you could eat chocolate cake all day and, as long as you're burning more calories than you're taking in, you'd still lose weight. But, there is such a thing as quality calories, and the more quality foods you eat, the more you'll get out of your meals and, consequently, the less calories you'll eat. There's also a connection between what you eat and how your body performs. If you eat a large, fatty meal and then try to exercise, you may find your energy level plummeting. Eating a more balanced meal can give your body the fuel it needs to operate at its best.

The foods you want to incorporate into your diet are nutrient dense, which means they offer more nutrients for fewer calories.

Whole grains, fruits, vegetables, and beans are considered nutrient dense because they can fill you up and keep you going with fewer calories. Foods that aren't nutrient dense (or what my clients often call "foods that are yummy") are often called empty-calorie foods and include things like sweets and sodas.

Nutrient-dense foods are what the USDA recommends you eat in their most recent *Dietary Guidelines*, published in 2005. These new guidelines also recommend:

- Eating a variety of foods and limiting our intake of saturated fat, trans fat, cholesterol, added sugar, salt, and alcohol
- Eating more dark green and orange veggies, beans, fruits, whole grains, and low-fat dairy products
- Eating a balanced diet based on the food-guide pyramid
- Choosing lean meats that can be baked, broiled, or grilled

The USDA also updated the food pyramid to help you figure out what and how much you should eat to stay healthy and lose weight. This new pyramid lays out the different food groups as well as daily recommended servings:

1. **Bread, cereal, rice, and pasta:** Eat at least 3 servings a day.
2. **Vegetables:** Eat at least 2–3 cups.
3. **Fruit:** Eat at least 2–3 cups.
4. **Milk:** Get at least 2.5–3 cups of fat-free or low-fat dairy products.
5. **Meat and beans:** Get at least 5–6 ounces of lean protein.
6. **Oil:** Get your oil from fish, nuts, and vegetable oils; avoid butter and shortening.
7. **Discretionary calories:** These foods might include naughtier choices like sweets or chips. The USDA recommends keeping these calories between 100 and 300.

ELSEWHERE ON THE WEB

▶ Understanding and using the food pyramid can be confusing. About.com's Nutrition Guide, Shereen Jegtvig, explains each part of the pyramid as well as the recommendations in her step-by-step guide to exploring the USDA food pyramid. This guide also includes helpful information about two other food pyramids that differ a bit from the USDA's version but offer other alternatives for creating a healthy diet. Visit http://about.com/nutrition/foodpyramid.

These recommended servings are just a rough estimate and can change according to your age, gender, and fitness level. To get a more personalized recommendation, visit MyPyramid.gov and enter in your information to get a list of each food group with recommended servings. The Web site also offers printable results, a meal-tracking worksheet, and a detailed assessment of your diet and physical activity.

One area that the food pyramid doesn't cover is how much water you should drink. Until recently, most of us have heard that we should drink at least eight glasses of water a day. But some reports have concluded that we can get adequate hydration by drinking when we're thirsty. We get water from a variety of sources, including milk, tea, juice, coffee, fruits, vegetables, and soda, just to name a few. To make sure you're staying hydrated, keep a water bottle handy and drink throughout the day. If your urine is clear, that's a good sign you're well hydrated.

If you're exercising, your fluid needs do change, and you want to make sure you're well hydrated before, during, and after your workouts. If you're dehydrated, your performance can suffer, and if you're exercising in extreme temperatures, being dehydrated can lead to nasty problems like heat exhaustion or, worse, heat stroke.

The guidelines for fluid replacement include drinking about two cups (or sixteen ounces) of water an hour before your workout and about four to eight ounces of water every fifteen minutes throughout your workout. Within thirty minutes after your workout, try to drink about sixteen to twenty-four ounces of water. If you find it hard to drink water during your workouts, try light sips every few minutes. If you exercise for more than an hour at a time, you may want to drink a sports drink to help you replace fluids and ensure you're getting rehydrated.

Now that you know all the guidelines for eating healthy, changing your diet should be fairly simple. The guidelines laid out by the USDA shouldn't come as a big surprise since most of us know we should eat more fruits and veggies and less sugary, fatty foods. The hard part is actually doing it, but there are a few simple ways to improve your diet by making small changes. Small changes may not mean huge results in the short term, but may mean long-term success. By changing your diet over time rather than all at once, those changes become permanent choices you can live with every day.

- **Add more fruit to your diet.** By adding something healthy, you can fill up on quality calories, leaving less room for the empty-calorie foods. Try adding it to your cereal, salads, or even your dinner.
- **Replace one unhealthy food every week.** Once a week, choose one unhealthy food you eat regularly and find a substitute that's healthier and has fewer calories. For example, instead of 2% milk, try 1% or skim.
- **Get your dressings and sauces on the side.** Whenever you order out, ask for any sauces or dressings to be served on the side so you can control how much you eat.
- **Sneak in more vegetables.** Pile your sandwiches with dark green lettuce and tomatoes, add spinach to your pasta dishes, and keep precut veggies handy for a healthy snack.

These are just a few suggestions for making small, lasting changes. What ideas can you come up with? Make a list and set a goal to tackle at least one thing on your list each week.

Should You Follow a Diet?

The food pyramid isn't the only game in town for changing your diet and losing weight. Another option is to do what millions of other people do each day and follow a specific diet. I'm not a big fan of diets, although I do think some of them can teach important lessons about eating healthy. The problem with many diets is that they're just too hard to follow, and people end up losing weight, then gaining it all back (and then some) when they go off the diet—which most people eventually do.

Some of the reasons diets don't work very well include:

TOOLS YOU NEED

▶ Most experts feel that effective and permanent weight loss happens by making lifestyle changes. While diets can help you lose weight temporarily, they often force you into programs that may not work for you rather than teaching you the Tools You Need to make those lifestyle changes. Eating healthy means working with your life as it is now. To learn more, check out my "Top 10 Reasons to Quit Dieting Forever" article at http://about.com/exercise/quitdieting and consider a different approach.

- **They're often hard to follow.** If you don't have a lot of time for grocery shopping and cooking every meal, following a diet for more than a few days or weeks may be impossible.
- **They're often unrealistic.** If you eat pasta every day and then follow a diet that banishes pasta completely from your diet, how long before you go on a pasta frenzy? Cutting out entire food groups is a sure way to make you want them even more.
- **They make you crazy ... and hungry.** Some diets are so restrictive or complicated, it's almost guaranteed you won't be able to follow them. Many fad diets (such as the Cabbage Soup Diet or the Grapefruit Diet) fall under this category.
- **They often don't fit with how you live.** If you eat out a lot or travel, you may not be able to follow the meal or menu plan set out by your diet.

This isn't to say that following a diet is always a bad idea or that you can't learn healthy eating tools from following diets. You just need to make sure the diet is reasonable, healthy, and fits with how you live. If you do decide to follow a diet, you'll want to follow a few basic tips for choosing a diet that's healthy and fits your lifestyle:

- Avoid quick-fix or fad diets that promise fast or guaranteed weight loss.

- Choose a diet that fits with your likes and dislikes. For example, if you hate meat, eggs, and dairy products, a low-carb diet may not be the best choice. Choose a diet that includes foods you enjoy and a plan you can see yourself following for the long term.
- Avoid diets that lower your calorie intake below 1,000 unless you're under a doctor's supervision.
- Choose a format that fits with your personality. If you need social support, a group like Weight Watchers might be a good choice for you. If you prefer a very structured approach, you might choose a diet that offers daily meal plans and recipes.
- Avoid diets that forbid specific food groups or include questionable supplements or drugs.

If you decide you'd like to follow a diet, your first step is to do some research. There are hundreds of diets out there, but you might start with the most common types of diets, such as low carb or low fat. Low-carb diets typically restrict the amount and/or type of carbs you can eat while increasing your protein intake and, in some cases, your fat intake as well. Atkins is a popular high-protein diet that allows for unlimited amounts of meat, cheese, and eggs while restricting carbs like sugar, bread, pasta, fruits, and veggies. Many people like Atkins because eating so much protein and fat can be satisfying, but you may find it hard to follow the Atkins Diet over the long term since carbs are so restricted. The downside is that the medical community is concerned about the effects of high amounts of protein and fat on the body and that nutrient-dense, high-fiber foods such as fruits and vegetables are restricted.

The Zone Diet is another popular lower-carb diet, which recommends you get 40 percent of your calories from carbs, 30 percent from protein, and 30 percent from fat. While the diet isn't as

▶ **Before you decide on a low-carb diet, take some time to figure out if this type of diet is right for you and what** *low carb* **really means. About.com's Low Carb Diets Guide, Laura Dolson, offers an excellent resource, "Getting Started on a** *Low Carb* **Diet," at** http://about. com/lowcarbdiets/getting- started, **explaining what** *low carb* **means and helping you figure out if it's the right kind of diet for you.**

restrictive as other diets and allows a broad range of food, experts worry that followers won't get the nutrients they need because it's such a low-calorie diet. The good thing about this diet is that it's easy to follow and it does encourage eating healthy, balanced meals.

Low-fat diets, which restrict the amount of fat you can eat, are also popular. One reason low-fat diets have been so popular is because we know that reducing fat is a simple way to cut calories. One gram of fat has 9 calories, as opposed to protein and carbs, which have 4 calories per gram. Cutting fat will naturally reduce your calorie intake if you don't add those calories somewhere else (fat also helps you feel satisfied, so if you lower your fat too much, you may eat more of other types of foods).

One of the popular low-fat diets is the Pritikin Diet, which encourages eating fruits, vegetables, and whole grains while restricting fat to about 10 percent of calories. While experts like the fact that this diet promotes healthy, balanced meals, they worry that the fat intake is too low. Dietary fat provides essential fatty acids the body may not get at these low levels.

Another popular diet is Weight Watchers, which stands out from the others because it isn't really a diet. Weight Watchers doesn't tell you what you can and can't eat, but instead, it gives you a daily points range and assigns point values to foods. You can eat what you want as long as you stay within your daily points range, and you can earn more points with exercise. Weight Watchers also includes group support meetings where members can meet on a regular basis for motivation and support.

Obviously, this doesn't cover every diet out there, but getting a feel for different types of diets, what they're all about and the pros and cons of each, can help you figure out which approach is right for you. Remember, any diet can work as long as you're restricting your calories, which is what most diets do.

Eating healthy can help you lose weight, but it can also have an effect on every other part of your life, including exercise. Eating a balanced diet can give you the energy your body needs to function at its peak, and you may find that if you start exercising regularly, you'll be more motivated to eat healthy. One healthy behavior often leads to another, and once you make the connection between what you eat and how you feel, you may start to look at food more as a fuel source than something to be obsessed about.

If you're exercising, one aspect of your diet to consider is when, how, and what you eat before and after your workouts. Getting the right nutrients beforehand will give you the energy you need for your workout, and eating the right foods after can help you repair and rebuild your body to keep you strong and healthy.

Some people find it hard to eat before a workout, especially if it's early in the morning. But your performance may suffer if you get hungry in the middle of your workout, so eating something light and easily digested (such as a yogurt or a banana) may be a good choice. The general recommendation is to eat a snack of about 200 to 300 calories, composed of mostly carbs and a moderate amount of fat and protein—fat and protein take longer to digest and may upset your stomach if you don't wait long enough to exercise after you eat. My favorite pre-workout snack is a small whole-grain bagel and a little low-fat yogurt.

It's important to eat something after your workout as well. There's a short window following your workout where your body works to repair damage and replenish some of the energy you used during your workout. By eating something within an hour after your workout, you can give your body the fuel it needs. The recommendations differ about what to eat after exercise, but the most common recommendation is to eat a snack that includes carbs and protein, such as a fruit smoothie or a protein shake.

The following are some general tips for eating and exercise:

- **Allow your body time to digest.** Large meals may require up to four hours, while smaller meals or snacks may require only one to three hours to digest.
- **Avoid exercising on an empty stomach.** It sometimes takes time to condition your body to handle food in the morning, but having even a little orange juice or a sports drink will give you more energy for your workout.
- **Avoid fatty foods before your workout.** Foods like meat, cheese, and other high-fat proteins take longer to digest and may leave you feeling tired during your workout.
- **Stay hydrated.** Being dehydrated can make you feel fatigued when you exercise.

You may find that it takes a little time and experimenting to find the right amount of food to eat and the right time to eat it. We're all different and may experience different rates of digestion, so don't be afraid to experiment with the guidelines to find what works for you.

Get Linked

The following resources at my **About.com** *Exercise site provide more insight into fueling your body in healthy ways for optimum performance and weight loss.*

NUTRITION FOR EXERCISE

Timing is everything when it comes to exercise and eating. This article provides more specific details for what and when to eat before and after your workouts.

 http://about.com/exercise/nutritionforexercise

THE TRUTH ABOUT LOW-CARB DIETS

Low-carb diets are popular, but some of these diets promote the idea that carbs can make you fat. While it's true that some types of carbs are better than others, that doesn't mean you should stop eating carbs completely. Learn more about what *low carb* really means in this article.

 http://about.com/exercise/lowcarbdiets

HOW MUCH PROTEIN DO YOU NEED?

Many low-carb diets promote higher protein as well. Meanwhile, the USDA says we already get plenty of protein every day. Who's right? Learn more about your protein needs in this article.

 http://about.com/exercise/protein

The **ABOUT**.com *Guide to* **Getting in Shape**

Chapter 11

Changing Your Program

Why Change Your Program?

One of the biggest mistakes I see beginner (and even advanced) exercisers make is doing the same thing for weeks, months, or even years. If you enjoy what you're doing and are happy with the results you're getting, you may be fine doing the same thing over and over. But if you've stopped seeing results and want to change your body, that means changing different elements of your program.

In previous chapters, you learned that one of the important aspects of exercise is overload. We often use that in terms of strength training, focusing on the idea that you need to lift weights that challenge your muscles. But the principle of overload applies to every part of your body and your exercise program. The great thing about the body is its ability to adapt to the stresses placed on it, and with exercise, the muscular and cardiovascular systems will usually adapt to your workouts within about four to eight weeks. Changing your program will help you reduce the risk of hitting a plateau, both mentally and physically.

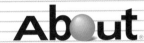

I'm worried that changing my routine will hurt my progress. What should I do?

▶ We're all creatures of habit, and those habits serve a purpose: helping us take care of our responsibilities. But being a slave to your workout routine is a sure way to get bored and burn out. Ask yourself which choice is better: changing your routine or continuing with the same old thing and eventually quitting altogether? Don't be afraid to break out!

There are some other problems you may experience if you do the same activities for too long, such as:

- **Repetitive stress injuries.** When you take your joints and connective tissue through the same motions day after day, you risk injuries or conditions such as tendonitis or bursitis.
- **Burnout.** Doing the same thing for too long can lead to disinterest or even a feeling of dread when thinking about your workouts.
- **Boredom.** Going to the gym and doing the same machines or walking the same route each day can leave you feeling uninspired and may make it hard to keep going.
- **Weight-loss or fitness plateaus.** When you don't continue to challenge your body with new activities, you may stop losing weight and/or seeing strength and endurance gains.

This means you have to change what you're doing, not just for your body to continue getting fit, but for your mind to stay interested in what you're doing. Nothing can turn you off of exercise faster than doing the same deadly dull program week after week. In fact, some studies have shown that exercisers who modify their routine every few weeks are more likely to stick with their programs.

Too often, people continue doing the same routine because they're afraid to change what they're doing. One reason may be that their workouts still feel difficult and challenging, even if the results are starting to wane. Another reason is fear of doing the wrong thing. What if you try something new and you don't burn the same number of calories or challenge yourself in the same way? Not only that, but you may be afraid that trying something new will make you quit. You've found a program you can follow—why mess with a good thing?

The good news is that you don't have to make major changes to continue seeing results, and those small changes can make you feel energized and help you recommit to your fitness goals with renewed enthusiasm.

If you're a beginner, it's important to stick with a routine and a program that works for you and allows you to condition your body, at least for a while. But at some point you'll need to change what you're doing, and there are some warning signs that it's time for a change:

- You start to dread your workouts.
- You realize you're finding excuses to skip workouts.
- You cut your workouts short because you're bored or uninterested.
- You start to miss more and more workouts.
- Workouts no longer feel challenging to you.

The following sections provide specific details for how to change your workouts, and the great news is, a little change goes a long way.

Add Variety to Your Current Workouts

If you're a beginner and you've been exercising for a few weeks, you may feel perfectly fine with the workouts you're doing. But remember, changing at least one aspect of your program every four to eight weeks can make a big difference in how an exercise or activity feels to you and, of course, how your body responds. Before we get into the details of making major changes in your workouts, there are some ways you can make simple changes to what you're doing right now. It involves manipulating different elements of your routine, such as your frequency, duration, and intensity.

ELSEWHERE ON THE WEB

▶ If your workouts seem boring, it's time to spice things up and take a few risks by breaking out of your exercise comfort zone. Jennifer R. Scott, About.com's Weight Loss Guide, helps you do that in her article "Variety … The Spice of Exercise." She discusses the importance of exercise variety in staying on track as well as specific things you can do to change your routine. Visit http://about.com/weightloss/variety.

One place to start is with your workout schedule. There are a number of ways to tweak your schedule either to allow more exercise time or to simply change what you're doing, which can open your mind to new possibilities. You may end up finding a new schedule you enjoy or a time of day that works better for you. Here are some ideas:

- **Change the number of days you exercise.** For example, you can add an extra day of cardio if you want more challenge, or simply shorten your usual workouts and spread them out over more days.
- **Change the order of your workouts.** Mixing things up from time to time can give you a fresh perspective on your workouts. Do strength training on the days you usually do cardio or vice versa, add an extra day of yoga or Pilates, or rest on a day you usually exercise.
- **Change when you exercise.** If you're a morning exerciser, try an afternoon or evening workout from time to time and vice versa. Workouts will feel different depending on when you do them, and you may find a new level of energy at a different time of the day.
- **Change the order of your exercises.** During a typical strength-training workout, start with the last exercise and work your way backward or jump around within your routine for a fresh approach.
- **Change where you work out.** If you usually go to the gym, try at least one outdoor or home workout every week or two. Without access to your usual machines, you may find new and creative ways to exercise.
- **Go faster for shorter workouts or go slower for longer workouts.** At least once every week or two, mix up the intensity of your workouts for a new challenge.

- **Change your route.** If you walk or jog outside, finding new and interesting places to go is essential for keeping both your mind and body interested. Try driving a few minutes away from your usual starting point and begin from a different street or trail.
- **Add 5 minutes of something new each week.** At the end of your workout, try 5 minutes of something different—a new gym machine; a run around the block; some kickboxing; or some strength moves like push-ups, squats, or crunches.

What other changes could you make to your current program to make it just a little different? Keep an exercise log and make a point to check in every week to determine what changes you could make to keep things interesting. Challenge yourself to make one small change each week.

How to Change Your Cardio Workouts

Now that you have some general ideas about workout changes, let's look at some specifics for your cardio workouts. In the cardio chapter, we discussed the different elements of a cardio workout: frequency, intensity, duration, and type of activity. By manipulating one or more of these elements, you can create new, challenging workouts to help you burn more calories and boost your endurance.

First, start with the frequency of your workouts and decide if it's something you'd like to change. Remember back in the first few chapters, we discussed exercise guidelines that dictate thirty to sixty minutes of exercise most days of the week. You can use that as a measuring stick against your own schedule and add more cardio to get closer to those guidelines, or you can go by what makes sense with your schedule. If you've hit a plateau or your workouts

WHAT'S HOT

▶ Now it's easier than ever to plan out a walking or running route and calculate your distance with Gmaps Pedometer (www.gmap-pedometer.com). There you can locate your city, click on the streets in your neighborhood, and record your route. You can measure the distance of each leg and get the total distance of your workout. Be warned: Planning out your routes can become addictive, and you may spend more time on the computer than on your walk!

are feeling a little too easy, adding a day of cardio is just one way to increase your calorie burn each week.

Another option, and even more of a challenge, is changing the intensity of your workouts. While it's true that adding intensity can make your workouts feel harder, you don't necessarily have to kill yourself to get the benefits, and you have a number of options for how to make your cardio workouts more intense. Even just working a little harder than usual can help you burn more calories and increase your endurance. Here are just some of the ways you can make cardio workouts more intense:

- **Go faster.** You can add speed to your workouts by either incorporating interval training (as discussed previously) or picking up the pace during your typical workouts so that you're working hard but still within your target heart-rate zone. You can do this for the entire workout or pick up the pace at different times throughout the workout.
- **Add resistance or incline.** If you're on a machine, you can work harder by increasing the resistance (as on a stationary bike or elliptical trainer), or you can raise the incline (as on a treadmill or an elliptical trainer with ramps). If you're outside, you can add more hills to your route.
- **Add upper-body moves.** Anytime you can involve both the upper and lower body, you can increase the intensity of your workouts. Try a cross-country ski machine, a VersaClimber, a rowing machine or just try swinging your arms on machines on which you usually hold on to the rails (like stair-steppers).

Another way to add intensity is to add some power moves to your workouts. A great way to do this is with plyometric exercises, or explosive moves that can get your heart rate up very high in a short period of time. Athletes often use plyometric training to enhance power, strength, and endurance for competition, but you don't have to train like an athlete to get the benefit of this type of training. In fact, a little bit goes a long way with power moves, and you should have several weeks of exercise under your belt before you incorporate plyometric training into your program. Some examples of these moves include:

- **Jumping from a grounded position.** This might be jumping up onto a low step or platform with both feet, stepping down, and repeating several times.
- **Squat jumps.** From a squat position, jump into the air and land back into a squat.
- **Lunge or scissor jumps.** From a lunge position, jump up into the air, switch legs, and land back into a lunge.
- **Power jacks.** These are like very slow jumping jacks—jump feet out wide and land in a squat, circling arms overhead. Jump feet back together and repeat.
- **Long jumps.** Start with feet together and squat while jumping forward as far as you can, landing in a squat, repeating several times.
- **Ski hops.** Start with feet together and lower into a squat. Jump to the side as far as you can, landing in a squat, then jump back to the other side.
- **Side-to-side jumps.** Leap to the right, landing on the right foot and cross the left arm diagonally in front of you. Jump to the left and repeat from side to side.

These are just a few examples of how to add a little power to your usual workouts, but you want to be careful how you use these moves. First, only add them once or twice a week, especially if you're a beginner. When adding these moves to your workouts,

TOOLS YOU NEED

▶ Adding power to your workouts is a great way to work up to your anaerobic threshold, a place where your body can get stronger and more enduring. By pushing yourself to new limits, you'll challenge your energy systems in new ways, burn more calories, and boost your endurance. But, it's important to be safe when doing plyometric exercises. To learn more about how to safely add more power to your workouts, check out my article "Hardcore Cardio," at http://about.com/exercise/hardcorecardio.

▶ Plyometric training isn't just for athletes. Home exercisers are finding more and more ways to add power to their workouts with exercise videos. Cathe Friedrich and Mindy Mylrea are just two video instructors who offer intense workouts, often using power moves in their step, kickboxing, boot camp, and hi/lo workouts. For some ideas, check out my Boot Camp Workout, which includes a variety of high-impact and power moves for a challenging workout. Visit http://about.com/exercise/bootcamp.

do each one for about 10 seconds and work your way up from there. These moves are high impact and can raise your heart rate very high, so take your time with them and stay within your own limits. These moves, when done too much or too hard, can cause injury, especially if you're a beginner or aren't used to high-impact activities, so be aware of that before trying them in your own workouts.

Some ideas for adding these power moves to your workouts include:

- Add one or two exercises throughout your normal work-out, repeating each one for ten or more seconds. For example, if you're walking outside, you could try ten long jumps every five or ten minutes.
- Add three to five minutes of power moves at the end of your workout; for example, try ten seconds each of squat jumps, power jacks, and ski hops; take a brief rest; and repeat one or more times.
- Do different power moves every two to three minutes of your workout; if you're doing a step workout, take a break every two minutes and try jumping onto the step with both feet or one foot at a time to raise your heart rate.
- Put them all together into a short, intense workout; for example, try each exercise listed for ten or more seconds, with a full minute (or more) of marching in place between each exercise to recover.

You can use these intensity ideas to change another element of your workouts: their duration. The power moves mentioned above are one way to add both time and intensity to a typical workout. You can also tweak the duration of your workouts by making them longer or shorter—just make sure you adjust the intensity accordingly. If you exercise for sixty minutes, you want to keep the intensity at a level you can sustain for the length of the workout, which might be a more moderate level. If you shorten your routine to thirty minutes, you may want to add intensity to get the most out of your time. Try a mix of workouts so you stay interested and work your body in different ways. The following workout schedule offers an example of a typical week for one of my clients, who enjoys step aerobics, running, and kickboxing:

Day 1 Rest

Day 2 Interval Step Workout—30 minutes (high intensity)

Day 3 Moderate Running—45 minutes (medium intensity)

Day 4 Rest or yoga

Day 5 Kickboxing Class—60 minutes (medium-high intensity)

Day 6 Rest or yoga

Day 7 Moderate Running—30 to 45 minutes (medium intensity)

For this client, each workout offers a different level of intensity for a different length of time so she doesn't get bored, and she gets an interesting mix of activities to keep her body challenged in a variety of ways.

Yet another way to change your cardio workouts is to try a different activity. In previous chapters, I've made suggestions to choose activities you enjoy, and that's exactly what you should do if you're a beginner. But as you get stronger, you'll want to branch out and allow your body and your muscles to work in different ways. Another name for this is **cross-training**, which simply means that your program involves a variety of different activities. When looking at your cardio workouts, make a note of what type of activity you usually do. Do you do the same activity for every workout? Is the activity usually low impact or high impact? Is it weight bearing or non–weight bearing? Categorizing your workouts can help you figure out gaps in your training where you could work your body in different ways. For example, if you're a swimmer, you're getting a great cardio workout, but it's not a weight-bearing activity. By adding something different (such as walking), you can strengthen your body in a way swimming can't. Use the following tips to determine what types of activities you could add to your routine to challenge yourself in different ways:

- If you usually do no- or low-impact activities such as the stationary bike or elliptical trainer, try something with impact, such as walking, running, a stair-stepper, or kickboxing.
- If you're a swimmer, try walking, cycling, or other weight-bearing exercises.
- If you always do intense, high-impact workouts, try something slower and gentler, such as a long bike ride.
- If you walk for exercise, try jogging, cycling, inline skating, or some other activity your body isn't so good at.
- If you tend to use the same cardio machine all the time, create a medley using different machines. For example, try ten minutes on the treadmill, ten minutes on the stair-stepper, and ten minutes on the stationary bike.
- If you exercise at home, create your own workout by turning on some music and doing your own moves. Try kicks, punches, or running up and down the stairs.

As an example of a cardio workout you could do at home in 10 minutes, try the following exercises, performing each for 30 seconds to 1 minute and modifying the high-impact moves if you need lower impact:

1. March in place or around the house, swinging the arms.
2. Jog in place or around the house.
3. High jogs: Bring the knees up to waist level if you can.
4. Jog or march in place.
5. Jumping jacks: Do 8 full jacks, 8 bringing the arms halfway up, and 8 starting with the arms up and bringing them halfway down.
6. Jump to the right, landing on right leg and swinging the left arm diagonally in front of you. Do the same to the left and repeat.
7. Jog or march in place.
8. High jogs: Bring the knees up to waist level.
9. Jumping jacks: Do 8 full jacks, 8 bringing the arms halfway up, and 8 starting with the arms up and bringing them halfway down.
10. March in place to cool down.

Setting New Goals

As you become more consistent with your exercise program, one thing you'll notice is that you're getting stronger, fitter, and faster. Not only that, but you may feel more confident—so confident that, after a while, you may want to try new and challenging activities. Part of changing your exercise program comes from that growing strength and confidence, which allows you to seek out new goals and new ways to exercise.

If you don't believe me, listen to this. Alice, a sixty-three-year-old client, was fairly active but starting to feel aches and pains she hadn't felt before. Alice stuck with the same walking and swimming workouts most of the time, but once we added strength training to her program, she saw some significant strength gains. She actually ended up training for and running in her first 5K, something she never thought she'd do.

ASK YOUR GUIDE

How do I know what to change about my cardio workouts?

▶ It's important to remember that you don't have to change everything at once. You might start by changing one thing each week, such as how often you exercise or how long your workouts are. For example, one week, try a new activity or machine. In two weeks, add five minutes of power moves to one of your workouts. In the next two weeks, add one extra day of cardio.

▶ **What many beginners don't know is that, by sticking with exercise, they can expect good things to happen. One thing you can expect is a greater appreciation for your body. Instead of looking at your flaws and imperfections, you'll start to feel your own strength and realize the amazing things your body does each day. To learn more about the good things in store for you, check out my article "Enjoying Exercise & Healthy Eating," at** http://about.com/exercise/ enjoy exercise.

Another client, Jane, had a different but even more powerful experience with exercise. She came to me as a Type-A go-getter who worked hard at everything she did, with no time for exercises that didn't challenge her in some way. I convinced her to come to a yoga class I was teaching, and though she had trouble relaxing during her first few classes, she ended up enjoying it so much that she actually created a yoga/meditation room in her house to help her relax and unwind. Giving herself permission to slow down made her realize that exercise isn't always just about burning calories.

As you can see, when starting an exercise program, you may end up doing things you never thought possible, and even better, your goals don't always have to be about doing something harder or faster or going farther. Your goals can also be about slowing down and incorporating other types of exercise into your program.

The key to setting new goals for yourself first begins with taking stock of where you are in your program. If you've been consistent with your cardio and strength training program for a few weeks, you might look at your old goals and see where you could make changes to further your progress or just make your exercise schedule work better for you. After about four to six weeks, sit down and look at different aspects of your workouts to see if you need to set new goals or make changes. Some examples might include:

● **How frequently you exercise.** Look back over the past few weeks and see how many workouts you've completed. If you've found it easy to stick with your schedule, consider making a small change such as adding another day of cardio or just a day of active rest (e.g., walking more throughout the day). If you've found it difficult to stick with the program, ask yourself if less frequent (or even more frequent) workouts would work better.

- **How long you exercise.** Are you able to fit in everything you need during your allotted workout time? Are your workouts too long or short? If so, you may need to change the duration of your workouts, either making them longer or shorter so you don't skip them.
- **How hard you're working.** Are your workouts still challenging to you? If not, you may need to speed up or add distance to your workouts. If you go by mileage, you could set a goal to go a little further each week. Just make sure you don't increase your mileage by more than 10 percent each week since more than that can cause injuries.
- **What type of exercise you're doing.** Do you like your workouts or do you just tolerate them? If they seem boring to you, think of new things to try or look for ways to enjoy what you're doing more (e.g., work out with a friend or download some new music to listen to).
- **Your workout schedule as a whole.** Does your schedule fit with your job, family, and social obligations, or do you find you skip workouts in favor of other tasks? Look for new ways to make exercise a priority for you whether that means a change of schedule or a change in your daily to-do list.

There are other ways to set new goals for yourself, especially if you're ready to take some risks and step out of your exercise comfort zone. One goal you might set is to try something completely different. What you choose will depend on what you've been doing and how far out you want to go. For example, if you've only worked out on the treadmill and machines at the gym, you might want to try a group fitness class. If you've only done cardio and strength training, you might try yoga, Pilates, or even belly dancing.

One favorite goal many of my clients like to set is training for a race. Entering a race or charity walk/run is an excellent way to move forward with your exercise while challenging yourself with something that will energize you in a whole different way. Some of the benefits of having a specific event to train for include:

ELSEWHERE ON THE WEB

▶ Training for a 5K race can take anywhere from a few weeks to a few months, depending on your fitness level. There are a number of great training programs out there, but your starting point should be About.com Running Guide Jesslyn Cumming's "Training Plans for Running a 5K," at http://about.com/running/5k. Here you'll find different training programs to fit all levels of fitness.

- **Motivation.** Training for a race is very specific. You'll have a strategy mapped out for each week and a specific date to shoot for, which can help motivate you to stick with your program each week.
- **Sense of accomplishment.** If you've never been in a race, entering one can be scary but exhilarating.
- **Competition.** If you're not usually competitive, running or walking in a race can energize you, forcing you to work harder than you would on your own.
- **Excitement.** Nothing matches the excitement and adrenaline rush of a race, and pushing your limits will help you realize what you're capable of.

There are a number of races you can choose from, such as 5K walks, 10K runs, a half marathon, or even a triathlon. If you're a beginner, a 5K is a great place to start because it's a reasonable distance (3.1 miles), and 5K races are often held all year round all around the country. There are also a number of mini-triathlons held throughout the year that are manageable for those of us who don't want to tackle iron-man distances. Danskin holds regular mini-triathlons for women throughout the country each year, and you can find more mini-triathlon races as well as other national races by visiting Active.com for information.

Another change you might need to make is your weight-loss goal. If you've been exercising for only a few weeks, you may not see significant results from your exercise and diet program. In fact, in my experience, most people don't start to see those changes until after three or more months of consistent exercise and healthy eating. If it's been only a few weeks, you might not want to change your goals, but if it's been a few months and you've gotten a feel for how quickly your body is changing, you may need to adjust your weight-loss goals to fit with what your body is actually doing.

Combining Workouts and Activities

Another way to change your program is to combine elements of different activities for a whole new type of workout. Think of this as the kitchen-sink approach where you throw in every exercise you can think of for a whole-body blast. This is a great choice if you're short on time and want to squeeze in everything from cardio and strength to yoga and flexibility. It's also great for shaking things up and pushing your body in different ways.

One example of this type of routine would be boot-camp workouts such as those mentioned previously in this chapter. Boot-camp workouts often combine strength-oriented moves like push-ups and crunches with cardio moves such as jumping jacks and squat-thrusts to help you build endurance and push past plateaus and boredom. This workout moves much like the circuit workouts discussed in previous chapters.

As an example of a boot-camp workout, try the following exercises, performing each for about 30 seconds to 2 minutes, depending on your fitness level, and modifying when needed. You can move through the exercises once for a shorter workout, or repeat them two or more times for a longer, more intense workout.

1. March in place or walk around the house to warm up
2. Jumping jacks
3. Crunches on the ball or floor
4. Pushups

5. Squat-thrusts. Squat down and place the hands on the floor. In an explosive move, jump up taking the legs back into a pushup position, then jump the legs back in and stand up, adding a jump at the end for more intensity.
6. Walking lunges
7. Close-grip pushups (with the hands under the shoulders)
8. Bicycle crunches
9. Mountain climbers. Begin in a pushup position with the right leg in and the left leg extended. Jump up and switch the feet in the air, bringing the left leg forward and the right leg back. Continue alternating legs as quickly as you can.
10. Side-to-side lunges

You can also combine other types of activities into your workouts. For example, you could set up a series of exercises that focus on cardio, lower-body strength, upper-body strength, Pilates, and yoga, moving through the same moves several times or creating a different series of movements. This example takes you through two series of movements:

1. 5 minutes on the elliptical trainer or treadmill
2. 16 reps of ball squats
3. 16 reps of pushups on the ball
4. Pilates exercise 100s
5. 30 seconds of the yoga poses downward facing dog and cobra

1. 5 minutes on the elliptical trainer or treadmill
2. 16 reps of walking lunges
3. 16 reps of bent over rows

4. Pilates double leg stretch
5. Yoga poses Warrior I, Warrior II, and Triangle pose, repeated on both sides

The key to combining activities is to throw out the rules and see how creative you can be with your workouts. For example, if you have twenty minutes for a workout, make a list of twenty exercises you could do, including everything from cardio and strength to flexibility and relaxation, and spend one minute doing each one. Or think of four different cardio activities and do each one for five minutes. Don't be afraid to throw together activities that focus on different areas of fitness. You may just find something new you enjoy.

Get Linked

The following resources at my About.com *Exercise site offer more tools to help you change your workouts and set new, exciting goals for yourself.*

BURN 300 CALORIES IN 30 MINUTES

This article describes specific ways you can change your workouts whether you use the treadmill, elliptical trainer, or stationary bike or do outdoor workouts.

 http://about.com/exercise/300calories

CARDIO BLAST WORKOUT

If you're looking for cardio exercises you can do at home, this Cardio Blast Workout provides some ideas for you. These high-impact moves can be done with no equipment and work best when done with your favorite music.

 http://about.com/exercise/cardioblast

6 WEEKS TO A HEALTHIER LIFESTYLE

If you'd like a more structured program to follow, consider signing up for this six-week course to help create a healthy lifestyle. Each week you'll receive a newsletter offering specific tips and workout ideas for making each day healthier than the one before.

 http://about.com/exercise/6weeks

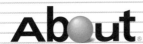

Chapter 12

How to Change Your Strength-Training Workouts

Changing Your Method of Training

In previous chapters, we talked about the need to change your program every four to eight weeks, and that also applies to your resistance-training program. You also learned about ways to set up a strength-training program such as total body workouts or split routines, which is one thing you can change when your workouts get a little too easy. But another way to change your workouts is by changing your method of training. Your training method is simply how you lift weights, and most of us start out with straight-set training, or performing a certain number of sets with rest in between. This is the most common method of training, but by no means is it your only choice. If you've been lifting weights for sev-

▶ Supersetting is a great choice if you want to save time in your workouts and increase the intensity at the same time. By working the same muscle group with different exercises, you can challenge your muscles without having to lift very heavy weights. For more benefits of supersetting and ideas for creating different types of workouts, check out my article "Quick Fix Workouts— Supersetting," at http://about. com/exercise/supersets.

eral weeks, you may want to try a different method of training to help strengthen your body in new and interesting ways.

One option is to do supersets. Supersetting involves doing two exercises for the same muscle group without resting, which means you're working harder but for shorter periods of time since you're not resting between sets. You can repeat each superset one or more times, depending on your goals, fitness level, and how much time you have. This is a good choice if you want a more challenging workout that can be done in a shorter period of time. The exercises below show some examples of supersets:

- Squats/leg extensions
- Deadlifts/hamstring curls
- Push-ups/chest presses
- Lat pulldowns/bent-over rows
- Overhead presses/lateral raises
- Barbell biceps curls/hammer curls
- Triceps dips/kickbacks

A more difficult training method involves tri-sets. This method involves performing three exercises for the same muscle group. As with supersetting, with this type of training, you'll perform all three exercises with very little rest between sets, which makes this a more advanced level of training. You can repeat each tri-set one to three times, depending on what your goals are and how much time you have. Some examples of this include:

- Squats/lunges/leg extensions
- Deadlifts/step-ups/hamstring curls
- Chest presses/push-ups/chest flies

- Bent-over rows/lat pulldowns/seated rows
- Front raises/lateral raises/reverse flies
- Barbell curls/hammer curls/concentration curls
- Triceps dips/triceps extensions/triceps pushdowns

You can also try working opposing muscle groups. With this type of training, one muscle rests while its opposing muscle contracts, which makes it a bit easier than supersets or tri-sets. Some examples include:

- Squat/deadlift
- Leg extension/hamstring curl
- Chest press/lat pulldown
- Front raise/reverse fly
- Biceps curl/triceps extension
- Crunch/back extension

Creating a push/pull workout split is another option. With this type of routine, which was discussed briefly in Chapter 5, you do mostly push exercises one day and concentrate on pulling exercises the next. Some typical push exercises include:

- Squats
- Leg extensions
- Push-ups
- Chest presses
- Overhead presses
- Triceps dips
- Calf raises

These pushing moves usually target the muscles of the quads, chest, shoulders, and triceps. Pulling exercises, on the other hand, often target different muscles, such as the back, hamstrings, and the biceps. Some examples of pulling exercises include:

- Deadlifts
- Hamstring curls
- Bent-over rows
- Lat pulldowns
- Upright rows
- Biceps curls

By using a push/pull routine, you'll be working different muscles during different workouts and can, therefore, lift weights more frequently.

If you want to lift heavier weights, a good way to ease into it is with pyramid training. With this training method, you progressively increase your weight and decrease your reps with each set. You can also work backward, decreasing your weight and increasing your reps with each set. An example of this type of training with a chest-press exercise would look like this:

Set 1   12 reps, 15 pounds
Set 2   10 reps, 20 pounds
Set 3   8 reps, 25 pounds

The key with pyramid training is to use enough weight for each set so that you can complete only the desired number of reps. This may take a little practice, so you may have to adjust your weights several times before you find what works for you. You can add even more intensity by pyramiding back up for a total of five sets.

▶ High-intensity strength training is one training method more exercisers are using to create challenging workouts. There are a number of ways to create high-intensity workouts, but one is to do ten reps of an exercise to fatigue, then reduce the weight 10 to 20 percent and complete three more reps. This type of training offers great results, but to avoid injury, you may want to do it for four weeks before going back to standard methods.

Trying New and Challenging Exercises

One of the simplest ways to change your strength-training work-outs is to try different exercises. Even if you're working the same muscle group, you'll immediately fire your muscle fibers in different ways, so it will feel like a whole new workout.

One option is to substitute exercises. For example, if you've been doing push-ups for your chest, switch to a chest press or fly. If you've been doing lat pulldowns for your back, try bent-over rows with a barbell or the assisted chin-up machine.

Another option is to change your position during the exercise, which can change how the exercise feels and involve different muscle groups to help you keep your balance. Some examples include:

- **Move from seated to standing.** For example, if you usually do an overhead press while seated, try it from a standing position.
- **Move from a regular stance to a split stance.** Even the simple act of changing where your feet are can make an exercise feel different. For example, stagger your feet during a biceps curl and you may find you use less momentum. Make a bent-over row more challenging by keeping the feet together instead of taking one leg back for support.
- **Stand on one leg.** Try standing on one leg while doing overhead presses or biceps curls and you'll add a balance challenge to your workouts.
- **Use one arm or one leg at a time.** This is one of my favorite ways to add challenge to workouts. Try one-legged squats and lunges or one-armed chest presses and flies and you'll notice how much harder you have to work to keep your balance. Just be sure to reduce your weights when switching from bilateral to unilateral moves.

TOOLS YOU NEED

▶ Circuit training is another way to change your work-outs and make them more interesting. Circuit train-ing means putting together several exercises and doing them one right after the other, rather than doing straight sets of the exercises. This type of training allows you to build strength and endurance with more variety. My Circuit Workout (http://about.com/exercise/circuit workout) includes compound strength-training moves that can be done in about thirty minutes for a short, challeng-ing workout.

- **Change your foundation.** This means changing what you stand or lie on during your exercises. For example, if you usually use a weight bench for chest presses or flies, try using an exercise ball. If you stand on the floor for squats, try them with one foot on an inflatable disc or other balance tool. Even resting one foot on a step or platform during standing exercises can change how your body moves and challenge you in different ways.

Another way to challenge yourself is by progressing with your exercises. Each strength-training exercise usually has several variations that allow you to start with a beginner move (such as chair squats or assisted lunges) and move on to more challenging moves (like free squats or forward lunges). By learning basic variations of standard strength moves, you can start to add more intensity to your workouts over time. Below, I've listed progression ideas, from easiest to hardest, for a few basic exercises:

Squats
1. Ball squats
2. Barbell or dumbbell squats
3. One-legged squats
4. One-legged squats on a BOSU or balance board

Lunges
1. Assisted lunge
2. Static lunge
3. Forward or reverse lunge
4. Walking lunge

ELSEWHERE ON THE WEB

▶ When changing position, you'll need some understanding of how best to target each muscle. When lifting weights, resistance needs to come from a certain direction to target the right muscles. For example, for a chest press to work, you need to be lying down. If you were standing, you'd work the shoulders rather than the chest. To learn more about how muscles work, check out the University of Michigan's "Hypermuscle: Muscles in Action," at www.med .umich.edu/lrc/Hypermuscle/ Hyper.html.

Push-ups

1. Wall push-ups
2. Push-ups on the knees
3. Push-ups on the toes
4. Push-ups with feet elevated on a step or ball

Chest Fly

1. Chest fly on the floor
2. Chest fly on a bench or step
3. Chest fly on the ball
4. One-armed chest fly on the ball

Crunches

1. Crunches on the floor, knees bent
2. Crunches with knees off the floor
3. Full crunches with both upper- and lower-body lifting
4. Bicycle crunches

Changing Reps, Sets, Weights, and Type of Resistance

Changing the number of reps and sets you do as well as the amount of weight you're using should top your list when it comes to changing your workouts. These types of changes can often be made every week, culminating in the larger changes (such as the training methods and exercise progressions discussed above) you'll make after four to eight weeks of training. For example, let's say you're starting out with a total body program that has you doing 1 set of each exercise for twelve reps. You might make the following changes on successive weeks:

▶ Progressing with your exercises simply means finding harder versions to try, whether you change the resistance you're using, try unilateral moves, or find different machines at the gym. You'll know you're ready to progress when an exercise feels easy to you. For a more complete chart of exercise progressions, visit my articles "Lower Body Progression" (http://about.com/exercise/lowerbodyprogress) and "Upper Body Progression" (http://about.com/exercise/upperbodyprogress).

Week 1 Add two reps per exercise (for a total 14 reps)

Week 2 Add a set (for a total of two sets)

Week 3 Add a set (for a total of two sets)

Week 4 Add weight per exercise (using enough that you can only complete 14 reps)

Week 5 Add two reps per exercise (for a total of 16 reps)

Week 6 Drop back down to 12 reps and increase the weight

Week 7 Add one more set (for a total of three sets)

Week 8 Change method of training to split upper- and lower-body routine

This example shows changes in all three areas: number of reps, number of sets, and the amount of weight you use. Remember, this is just one example and not the only way to progress in your workouts each week. In fact, once you've been strength training for a while, you may find you want to change your workouts every four weeks or more frequently. Many of my clients have been exercising for long enough that I often change their workouts every week for variety, which is another option if you're experienced and can handle different exercises from week to week.

Changing the type of resistance you use is another way to change what you're doing and add a new dimension to your training. If you usually use machines, switch to free weights or vice versa. If you've never tried the cable machine, try some of your exercises there. For example, instead of a chest press on the machine, try a one-armed cable press or a cross-over chest fly. Another interesting option is to fuse different types of resistance together, such as holding dumb-bells while using a resistance band for different exercises.

Obviously, there are a number of ways to change your workouts and it may seem overwhelming at first. But remember, you don't have to change everything at once. Choose just one of the options and you're on the right track.

The following tables show one workout taken through three phases of a total body exercise program, each phase lasting four weeks and showing a progression of sets, weights, reps, and/or exercises.

PHASE I: TOTAL BODY

Exercise	Week 1	Week 2	Week 3	Week 4
Machine chest press	1 × 12	2 × 12, add weight	2 × 14	2 × 12, add weight
Lat pulldown machine	1 × 12	2 × 12, add weight	2 × 14	2 × 12, add weight
Seated overhead press	1 × 12	2 × 12, add weight	2 × 14	2 × 12, add weight
Dumbbell bicep curls	1 × 12	2 × 12, add weight	2 × 14	2 × 12, add weight
Triceps pushdowns	1 × 12	2 × 12, add weight	2 × 14	2 × 12, add weight
Leg press	1 × 12	2 × 12, add weight	2 × 14	2 × 12, add weight
Chair squats	1 × 12	2 × 12, add weight	2 × 14	2 × 12, add weight
Assisted lunges	1 × 12	2 × 12, add weight	2 × 14	2 × 12, add weight
Crunches	1 × 12	2 × 12	2 × 14	3 × 14
Back extensions	1 × 12	2 × 12	2 × 14	3 × 14

Exercise	Week 1	Week 2	Week 3	Week 4
Chest press	2 × 12	2 × 12, add weight	3 × 12	3 × 12, add weight
Push-ups on knees	2 × 12	2 × 12	3 × 12	3 × 12
Lat pulldown/ reverse grip	2 × 12	2 × 12, add weight	3 × 12	3 × 12, add weight
Bent-over rows	2 × 12	2 × 12, add weight	3 × 12	3 × 12, add weight
Reverse fly	2 × 12	2 × 12, add weight	2 × 14	2 × 14, add weight
Standing overhead press	2 × 12	2 × 12, add weight	2 × 14	2 × 14, add weight
Barbell biceps curls	2 × 12	2 × 12, add weight	2 × 14	2 × 14, add weight
One-armed triceps pushdown	2 × 12	2 × 12, add weight	2 × 14	2 × 14, add weight
One-legged leg press	2 × 12	2 × 12, add weight	2 × 14	2 × 12, add weight
Squats with dumbbells	2 × 12	2 × 12, add weight	3 × 14	3 × 12, add weight
Lunges	2 × 12	2 × 12, add weight	2 × 14	2 × 14, add weight
Ball crunches	2 × 12	2 × 14	2 × 16	3 × 16
Back extensions on the ball	2 × 12	2 × 14	2 × 16	3 × 16

Exercise	Week 1	Week 2	Week 3	Week 4
Incline chest press	3 × 12	3 × 14	3 × 16	3 × 12, add weight
One-armed chest fly	2 × 12	2 × 14	2 × 16	2 × 12, add weight
Push-ups on toes	1 × 12	2 × 12	2 × 14	2 × 16
Dumbbell pullover	3 × 12	3 × 14	3 × 16	3 × 12, add weight
One-armed reverse fly	2 × 10	2 × 12	2 × 14	2 × 10, add weight
One-armed overhead press	2 × 10	2 × 12	2 × 14	2 × 10, add weight
Lateral raises add weight	2 × 12	2 × 14	2 × 16	2 × 12
Cable biceps curls	2 × 12	2 × 14	2 × 16	2 × 12, add weight
Concentration curls	2 × 12	2 × 14	2 × 16	2 × 12, add weight
Triceps dips	2 × 12	2 × 14	2 × 16	2 × 12, take feet farther out
Triceps extensions	2 × 12	2 × 14	2 × 16	2 × 12, add weight
Barbell squats	3 × 12	3 × 14	3 × 16	3 × 12, add weight
Walking lunges	3 × 12	3 × 14	3 × 16	3 × 12, add weight
Barbell deadlifts	3 × 12	3 × 14	3 × 16	3 × 12, add weight

Exercise	Week 1	Week 2	Week 3	Week 4
Hamstring rolls	2 × 12	2 × 14	2 × 16	2 × 12, one leg at a time
Ball crunches	2 × 12	2 × 14	2 × 16	2 × 16
Knee tucks	2 × 12	2 × 14	2 × 16	2 × 16
Back extension on the ball	2 × 12	2 × 14	2 × 16	2 × 16

Tools to Add Challenge and Variety

One of the most interesting ways to add variety and challenge to your workouts is to use some of the new balancing tools that are becoming more and more popular. The exercise ball is one such tool, and you've learned a number of ways to use it for strength and flexibility. But another hot piece of equipment is the BOSU Balance Trainer.

The BOSU (an acronym for "both sides up") Balance Trainer is almost like an exercise ball that's been cut in half, with a platform placed on the bottom so you can use the dome side or the platform side for a variety of exercises. The BOSU Balance Trainer can be used for cardio, strength, and even yoga, Pilates, and flexibility exercises, and best of all, it adds an element of fun to your workouts.

For cardio, you can use the BOSU Balance Trainer almost like a step, performing step-ups, straddle-steps, and jumping moves like squats or lunges off the side. You can stand on it to add a balance challenge for everything from squats and biceps curls to overhead presses and lateral raises. By simply standing on it while performing traditional exercises, you can create a dynamic environment that requires all your concentration and stability muscles to keep you on top.

The BOSU Balance Trainer is also an excellent tool to strengthen the core. You can sit on it and perform ab exercises like V-sits,

▶ The BOSU Balance Trainer is an excellent addition to your home gym if you're looking for something fun and challenging. You may also find different types of BOSU classes at your local health club or gym. To learn more about the BOSU Balance Trainer, where you can buy it, and different exercises you can try, check out my article "The BOSU Balance Trainer," at http://about.com/exercise/bosu.

crunches, and oblique curls. You can lie on your side for challenging oblique work or use it on all fours with your knees on top for difficult balancing moves. It can also be used like a weight bench, supporting your head and neck for exercises like chest presses, flies, triceps extensions, and pullovers. Because you're in a bridge position (with the hips lifted), you get the lower body and the core involved in every exercise.

With the platform side up you can do plank exercises while rocking the BOSU back and forth, and you can also do a variety of push-ups and yoga moves like downward dog, forward lunges, and more. There are a variety of BOSU Balance Trainer videos and DVDs available at Bosu.com (www.bosu.com).

Another interesting new tool is the Gliding Sliding Disc Exercise System (or Gliders), available at GlidingDiscs.com (http://gliding discs.com). These are flat plastic discs about the size of paper plates that allow you to slide during different exercises so you incorporate a variety of muscle groups. At about $16 a pair, they're very affordable and you can do a number of exercises. Place a Glider under one foot and slide it back into a lunge. By pressing the foot into the Glider and pulling it back, you'll involve more quad muscles of the back leg as well as your core. You can also use them for side and diagonal lunges, standing leg circles, and even for challenging ab work and chest work. By placing a disc under each hand, you can slide the hands out as you lower into a push-up and slide them back together as you come up, which will involve more muscle fibers.

Foam rollers are another tool making their way from the world of physical therapy into the world of fitness. These can be used for balance training, core work, and flexibility exercises, and you can even roll on them with different areas of the body to help massage tight muscles.

ASK YOUR GUIDE

I've seen foam rollers, but how do I use them in my workouts?

▶ Foam rollers can be used to support your back during ab exercises or, if you lie on the roller horizontally, to challenge you during crunches or leg lifts. Position your hands on it for push-ups, which adds instability, or you can use a half-roller to stand on for squats, lunges, and other lower-body exercises. For more, check out my "Strength and Stretch with the FitBALL Roller" article at http://about.com/ exercise/ fitball.

Other Ways to Spice Up Your Workouts

If trying to figure out how to change your workouts is confusing or you can't seem to get out of the same old routine, it may be time to break out and try something completely different. Hiring a personal trainer is just one way to do this. In previous chapters I've discussed reasons you may want to hire a personal trainer to help you set up your exercise program. While beginners can get a lot out of working with a trainer or some other type of fitness expert, more advanced exercisers often get more out the experience because they already know the basics of exercise and have the strength to go further and do more.

If you've been exercising for a while and are running out of ideas, a trainer can be an excellent choice for getting out of your rut. A trainer can:

- Help you tweak your form to get the most out of the exercises
- Push you to work harder
- Come up with new and challenging exercises
- Offer new ideas for fitness goals
- Create innovative workouts to keep both your mind and body challenged

And don't forget, as mentioned back in Chapter 2, you can also try online training if hiring a personal trainer is out of your budget or doesn't fit with your schedule. With online training you can print your workouts and do them anywhere, anytime, giving you complete control over your exercise time.

Taking a group fitness class is another way to bring new life to your strength workouts. By ditching the solo workouts and joining a group strength class at the gym, you not only engage in different types of workouts with new equipment, you can also feed off the group energy you often don't get when training alone. Group strength training is a great way to get support and stir up your competitive juices to make your strength workouts a little less dull.

Get Linked

The following resources at my **About.com** *Exercise site offer more ideas for how to change your strength-training workouts as well as make the best use of your time for weight loss and strength gains.*

GET OUT OF YOUR RUT

This article offers even more ideas for changing your method of training, from eccentric work and forced reps to pre-exhaustion and circuits.

 http://about.com/exercise/rut

GETTING THE MOST OUT OF STRENGTH TRAINING

You learned about different ways to change your exercises so that they're more challenging for you, and this article describes even more ideas for you to try.

 http://about.com/exercise/mostofstrength

TOTAL BODY STRENGTH, BALANCE, AND STABILITY

This workout offers a total body program to make you stronger, to to improve your balance, and to involve more muscles to keep you stable. This is a great workout to try if you need some variety and are ready for a challenge.

 http://about.com/exercise/totalstrength

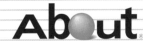

Chapter 13

Avoiding Plateaus and Staying Motivated

Understanding Plateaus

The previous chapters have given you some ideas for how to change your workouts to keep things fresh, interesting, and, of course, to avoid hitting weight loss or strength plateaus. Plateaus are normal and happen to everyone whether you've been exercising for years or for just a few weeks. In fact, even if you do make small changes in your exercise program, that may not be enough to stop your body from hitting a plateau. Learning more about why and how plateaus happen and how to handle them is important for keeping you on track with your exercise program.

Exercise plateaus can come from a number of directions. Maybe you've stopped seeing strength gains or you're no longer losing fat as quickly as you were before. Some people find they hit an endurance plateau and that no matter how hard they try, they can't seem to go faster or reach a certain distance. Hitting a wall with your training could mean that you've reached your body's limits, but more likely, it means you've hit a wall with your training or your diet (or both) and simply need to make some changes to keep seeing results.

What if you're not losing weight? One thing that happens when you start exercising and eating healthy is that your body changes. You lose body fat, you start to see more muscles, and you may have to go out and buy new clothes to fit your new, svelte shape. The problem is those changes can lead to slower weight loss. Most people will experience a slowdown in their weight loss after some initial progress, even though they're still exercising and following a healthy diet. The reason? The less you weigh, the less energy it takes to move your body. So a person who is 100 pounds overweight will lose weight faster than a person who is only 10 pounds overweight.

If you've hit a plateau, it's important to look at each element of your diet and program to make sure your program is balanced and that you're eating healthy, balanced meals. First, make sure you're eating enough calories so that your body can function while still losing weight. Back in the chapter on nutrition, we talked about the problems that can happen when you lower your calories too much—your body may go into starvation mode if it isn't getting enough fuel. If you're skipping meals or eating very little throughout the day, you may see your weight loss slow down.

Second, make sure you're not losing muscle along with the fat. Muscle is more metabolically active, so the more muscle you have, the more calories you'll burn all day long. If you're lifting weights regularly, you probably don't have to worry about this, but if you're doing only cardio, you risk losing muscle along with the fat, which can slow weight loss.

TOOLS YOU NEED

▶ There are a number of factors involved in weight loss, many of which are out of our control (think genetics, hormones, and aging). But there are a number of things you can control, such as your eating, how much exercise you get, and how you handle your stress. My article "10 Reasons You're Not Losing Weight" discusses the most common reasons for plateaus and what you can do about them. Visit http://about.com/exercise/notlosingweight.

Third, make sure you're changing your program every four to eight weeks. The previous chapters discussed a variety of ways to change what you're doing every few weeks—make sure you continue challenging your body with new exercises and workouts as your body adapts and becomes more efficient at exercise. Remember, even small changes help, so don't feel that you have to recreate a whole new routine every week if that's something you wouldn't enjoy.

If you're doing all of the above and the weight still isn't budging, the first place to look is at your diet. If you've been tracking your calories as you've been losing weight, have you gone back to recalculate a new BMR based on your new weight? Remember, as you lose weight, your body will require fewer calories, so you need to adjust those calories throughout the weight-loss process. For example, if you are a thirty-five-year-old female who is five foot seven and weighs 155 pounds, your BMR would be about 1,480 calories. If you lost 20 pounds, your BMR drops to 1,392—an 88-calorie difference. This may not seem like much, but if you ate an extra 88 calories every day for a year, you'd gain almost 10 pounds. This is something most people don't take into account and one reason for weight-loss plateaus.

Another factor to look at if you've hit a plateau is overtraining. Doing too much exercise can be just as bad as not doing enough. If you increase your intensity too much, your body may respond by decreasing the number of calories you burn the rest of the day. You'll learn more about the signs of overtraining in the next chapter, but the idea is to ease into an exercise program when you're just starting out and allow your body time to rest and recover.

Another less common cause of plateaus is a medical condition such as a problem with your thyroid. A thyroid deficiency can slow metabolism, which may lead to weight gain even though you haven't changed your diet or your exercise program. Only your

▶ Thyroid diseases affect millions of people and can cause problems in every area of health, not just weight gain. The problem is, they're often difficult to diagnose. About.com's Thyroid Disease Guide, Mary Shomon, suspects that there are millions of people walking around with undiagnosed thyroid problems. To learn about the causes and symptoms of thyroid diseases, check out her article "Thyroid Disease 101," at http://about.com/thyroid/thyroid101.

doctor can diagnose thyroid problems, and you should see your doctor if you've noticed any unexplained weight gain. Keep in mind that some medications can cause weight gain as well, especially some birth control medications, antidepressants, and diabetes medications. Always ask your doctor about that to learn if weight gain might be a side effect of any drugs you're taking.

If you've gone through these different scenarios and are following all the rules, one last thing to look at is this: success! It isn't unusual for people to set weight-loss goals that are a little lower than what works best for their bodies and lifestyles. You'll often hear these people talking about losing those last few pounds. If you've been trying to lose those last 5 or 10 pounds for more than a few months and you're just not able to get there, it might be time to let go of that goal and decide that where you are is just fine. It may be that you could exercise more and eat less to lose that weight, but if your current diet and program are working for you, you may not feel very motivated to do that. In fact, I don't know a single person, no matter how much they weigh, who doesn't want to lose at least a few pounds!

If your doctor says you need to lose weight for your health, that's a good reason to continue working past that plateau. But if you're in a healthy weight range, consider moving on to goals other than weight loss. It may be that focusing your attention on something new and challenging will end up helping you lose those extra pounds without even trying.

Worse than hitting a weight-loss plateau is realizing you're gaining weight. This is another common problem beginners often experience, and as with weight-loss plateaus, there are a number of reasons you could be gaining weight.

First, you should determine if you're really gaining fat (and getting bigger) or if you're gaining muscle (and slimming down). If you're going only by the number on the scale, that number can be deceiving. Muscle is denser than fat, so if you gain a little muscle, the scale could go up. But muscle also takes up less space than fat, so your body may be slimming down. If you're losing inches and your clothes feel a bit looser in different areas, forget about the number on the scale because you're on the right track.

If you decide that you are gaining weight and getting bigger, the first place to look is at what you're eating. Your diet is the most crucial component in the journey to weight loss, and many of us underestimate the importance of what we're eating. In my experience, most weight-loss problems are the result of what my clients are eating, more than the exercise they're doing, because it's very easy to take in extra calories without even realizing it. This is when keeping a food journal becomes essential. Some things to look at with your diet may be:

- **Liquid calories.** Many people forget to count the beverages they're drinking. For example, drinking a lot of fruit juice or sports drinks can add extra calories, and visiting coffee shops on a regular basis for smoothies and other sweet drinks can pile on more calories than you think.
- **Alcohol consumption.** This is another area where many of us don't keep track of extra calories. On the average, twelve ounces of light beer can contain more than 100 calories—drink four or five of those in one sitting and you've taken in an extra 400 to 500 calories.
- **Hidden calories.** Do you put a lot of cream in your coffee? Do you nibble on snacks throughout the day that you don't keep track of? Write down every single thing you eat, even if it comes down to counting peanuts or chips to make sure you really are eating the calories you think you are.

ASK YOUR GUIDE

I've been exercising hard for almost a month, so why am I not seeing results?

▶ Weight loss takes time, and your body doesn't always respond to exercise immediately. For most people, the body may need time to adjust to your new exercise program and eating habits, so you won't necessarily see any immediate weight loss. Give yourself two or three months with your program before you give up or decide you're doing something wrong.

▶ Making healthy meals
seems like a lot of work, but
the latest frozen meals make
healthy eating a snap. If you
don't have time to cook,
frozen meals can be a good
choice since the calories are
counted for you, and if you
choose wisely, you'll get a
balanced meal that tastes
pretty good. Experts rec-
ommend you choose meals
that are low in calories (less
than 300) and salt and that
contain vegetables and whole
grains.

- **Measure, measure, measure.** Many of my clients complain about having to measure their food, but they're always shocked when they actually do it and see how much they're really eating. Measure everything you eat for one week to see if you're on track.
- **Making your own meals.** The only way to really know what's in your food is to make it yourself. Eating out, even if you choose healthier options, can lead to eating more calories.

Another reason you may be gaining weight is that you could be gaining muscle faster than you're losing fat. We all have different body types, muscle fibers, and genes, and for that reason, our bodies will often respond to exercise in different ways. Some people may find they build muscle more quickly, and if they aren't losing fat quite as fast, they may experience an initial weight gain. If that's the case for you, don't panic and quit your program. Instead, either allow your body time to respond to what you're doing, or tweak your program to ensure you're getting enough cardio along with your strength training. You don't want to stop lifting weights, but you may want to shift your focus to muscular endurance (for example, keeping your reps between 12 and 16 with a lighter weight) rather than strength (for example, 8 to 12 reps with a heavier weight).

Staying Motivated

Plateaus don't just happen to your body, they can also happen to your mind. I once showed up at a client's house for a session only to find her sprawled on the treadmill, an arm flung over her eyes. "I *loathe* this treadmill," she said when I asked her what was wrong. "In fact, if I have to work out in this room for one more moment, I'll probably die." While she tended toward the dramatic, I knew exactly how she felt, having experienced that feeling in my own workouts. I knew if we didn't find some way to keep her motivated, she would probably quit exercising.

The thing about motivation is that it's something you have to work on each day. Many people wait to feel motivated, thinking if they just wait long enough, they'll wake up one day excited to exercise. But unfortunately, it doesn't work that way. In fact, motivation is just the opposite—you have to create it, and even more important, you have to re-create it each and every day.

Motivation can come from anywhere, and you may find what motivates you one day won't work the next. The key is to keep working to find something to get you out the door if that first idea doesn't work. The first place to start is with your goals. If you're exercising, there's a reason you're doing it. You may want to lose weight, get fit, deal with a health issue, or just feel better about yourself. Whatever your goal is, focusing on it is a great way to stay on track with exercise. Write down your goal (or cut out a picture of what your goal looks like) and put it on the fridge, the steering wheel of your car, your computer—anyplace that's visible to you on a regular basis. Sometimes just seeing that goal in black and white will be enough to keep you moving.

Of course, there will be times when your goal seems so far away, it doesn't have enough oomph to get past your reluctance to exercise. If focusing on your goals isn't working, rely on your self-discipline. Sometimes you work out simply because it's part of your schedule and you promised yourself you'd do it. Following through will allow you to trust yourself to keep your commitments, even when times get tough.

Inspiration is another great way to motivate yourself. Think of someone you look up to, someone who takes care of himself and exercises on a regular basis, even when he doesn't feel like it. Picture that person exercising and then visualize yourself going through your own workout. You may find that just imagining your

ELSEWHERE ON THE WEB

▶ Motivation seems like a hard thing to come by some days, and most of us struggle to be healthy on a regular basis. But it's nice to know you're not alone, and one way to get motivated is to learn what other people do to stay on track. Mary Shomon, About.com's Thyroid Disease Guide, offers tips for staying motivated in her article "How to Keep Exercising and Keep It Exciting!" at http://about.com/thyroid/exercisetips.

success is enough to get you going. When I don't feel like exercising, I always think of my grandmother who is in her eighties and goes to water aerobics twice a week, no matter how she's feeling. If she can exercise, there's no reason I can't exercise, too.

Another way to motivate yourself is by stirring up your competitive juices. If you're thinking of skipping your workout, just imagine all the other people who are exercising right now. Picture them streaming into gyms and walking down sidewalks all over the world, sweating and working and getting fit. Don't let them beat you! If they can make it to their workout, so can you. Or you could train for a charity race, as mentioned in previous chapters. Having something specific to work for always makes exercise a little easier.

Having a workout buddy can be a great motivator as well, as can working with a personal trainer. Having an appointment with someone else helps make exercise more of a priority, and if that still doesn't get you moving, try a good old-fashioned bribe. Promise yourself that if you exercise for ten minutes and still don't want to keep going, you can quit and go home. Most of the time, you'll want to keep going.

Another way to get yourself moving is to think about what this workout might mean for your future. Each workout you do is essential to your goals to lose weight, get healthy, and have a better quality of life. Remind yourself that this workout has a direct effect on whether you reach your goals sooner rather than later.

When and How to Take a Break

Remember the client I mentioned in the previous section? The one who felt she would die if she had to do one more workout? After some discussion, we both came to the conclusion that she needed a break from her routine. In her case, she'd been doing strength training and cardio workouts and, though we changed her program

WHAT'S HOT

▶ The fitness industry has a lot going on, working hard to help American adults and kids get healthy. To that end, the IDEA Health & Fitness Association has launched Inspire the World to Fitness, an initiative designed to bring fitness professionals together to help combat America's weight problem. Through this initiative, IDEA is challenging fitness pros all over the country to inspire five new people to start exercising each year. Could you be one of them?

often, she was simply burned out doing the same old thing. To get her back on track, she took an entire week off from exercise, and when she came back, we started a new program with different activities.

Sometimes, you need a break from structured exercise, especially if you've been following the same schedule for a while and are starting to feel a little burned out. For some exercisers, it's tough to take a break since the phrase "use it or lose it" is at the heart of exercise. If you stop exercising for too long, you can lose all the strength and endurance gains you've made. But a break can be worth it if it leaves you feeling rested and rejuvenated when you get back to exercise.

So, the question becomes, how fast do you lose it if you take a break from exercise? If you take a break for one week, your cardio fitness can decline about 5 percent, depending on how fit you were to begin with. In two weeks you'll lose about 15 percent, and up to 25 percent in three weeks, so taking a week off shouldn't significantly affect your endurance. Your muscle mass and strength will often take longer to decline, but experts recommend taking no more than a week off to avoid losing that strength.

If you reach a point where you feel burned out and tired of the same old thing, it may be time to plan a break. Planning it in advance gives you something to look forward to and helps you avoid getting to a point where you hate what you're doing so much you feel like quitting permanently. And you don't necessarily have to stop exercising completely, if being inactive worries you. Here are a few ways you can take some time off:

- **Take time off from everything.** In most cases, this would mean taking an entire week off from all structured exercise, though you might continue with light, more spontaneous activities.

What should I do if I have a hard time taking a break from exercise?

▶ While some of us struggle to exercise, there are others who have a hard time taking a break, even when they need it. Like anything else, exercise can become an obsession. If exercise is taking over your life or you become depressed when you have to miss a workout, you may need to see your doctor or therapist to help you deal with other issues.

- **Take an active rest.** This simply means staying active with activities outside of your program. An active rest might be a good choice if you're spending a week moving (lifting and carrying boxes for hours on end is a workout in itself) or building something or are involved in some type of physical project where you don't have time for exercise.
- **Try completely different activities.** In this case, you might trade your usual routine for something new—swimming instead of running, or walking outside instead of going to the gym. Try a belly-dancing class instead of ab exercises or play tag with your kids instead of an interval workout on the treadmill.
- **Take a week to shift your focus.** If you usually do hard, intense workouts, you might take a week to try only slow, gentle workouts like stretching or yoga. If you usually do more cardio workouts, try just strength training for a week or vice versa.

Of course, there can be drawbacks to taking a break from exercise, especially if you're a beginner. Many beginners need continuous exercise for a while to keep them on track. Some newbies find that taking two or three days off often leads to weeks or months without exercise, so you may need to be a bit strict with yourself at first and then ease off when you know you can trust yourself to get back to your program.

Keeping Exercise a Priority

Part of staying motivated and being consistent with your workouts is making exercise a priority. That means your workout time should be just as important as work, family obligations, and anything else you do each day. The reality is that, if we don't get our exercise in first thing, it usually ends up at the bottom of our to-do lists. There are a number of reasons that exercise loses importance for us, and one main reason is unrealistic expectations. When we expect to get something out of our workout program and it doesn't happen, it's easy to skip exercise since it doesn't seem to give us what we want. Take a look at the following list to see if any of these unrealistic expectations resonate with you:

- You expect to lose weight immediately.
- You expect exercise to be temporary.
- You expect to feel motivated to exercise each day.
- You expect major changes in your body.
- You expect exercise to be easy.

Having these kinds of expectations and then realizing they aren't going to happen (or at least not on your timetable) can lead to disappointment, disillusionment, and a general feeling of why-bother-itis. Why bother doing your workout if you aren't going to see immediate results? Part of keeping exercise a priority is getting rid of these unrealistic expectations and recommitting to exercise—not just for the physical changes you want, but for better health and quality of life.

If you skip more workouts than you end up doing, stop and ask what you really want for yourself. Too often we talk about things we want but don't do anything to get them. If you want to lose weight and you're not doing the exercise you need to reach that goal, ask yourself if losing weight is really something you want for yourself. If you wanted it, wouldn't you be working for it?

Take some time to think about past successes, goals you set for yourself and reached. Maybe you got a college degree or went through extra training for a promotion at work. Thinking about it, you probably have a number of successes under your belt, so there's no question you know how to reach a goal. The trick is finding a goal you really want to reach and realizing that losing weight may

TOOLS YOU NEED

▶ If you do find you've ended up taking a break that's a little longer than you planned, don't panic! It takes practice to get into a consistent exercise routine, and it's normal to experience failure from time to time. In my article "The Right Way to Fail at Exercise," I discuss some of the common reasons we fail and why failure isn't always such a bad thing. Visit http://about.com/exercise/rightway tofail.

not be that goal. That doesn't mean you give up on exercise or even give up on the idea of changing your body; what it does mean is setting a goal you feel strongly about and that is meaningful for you. If it means something, you'll make it a priority.

Get Linked

The following resources at my **About.com** *Exercise site will teach you how to motivate yourself and give you ideas for what you can do to stay on track with your exercise program.*

5 WAYS TO STICK WITH YOUR EXERCISE GOALS

In order to have some staying power with your workout program, you may need to have a few tricks up your sleeve. This article discusses five things you can do to make exercise a little easier.

 http://about.com/exercise/stickwithgoals

GETTING MOTIVATED TO EXERCISE

This article delves into the idea of motivation and helps you redefine what it means to you. Learn about what makes you tick so you can keep going with your exercise routine.

 http://about.com/exercise/motivated

STAYING COMMITTED TO EXERCISE

Staying committed to your exercise program is a lot like staying committed to a long-term relationship. There has to be some nurturing, a little compromise, and a lot of trust. Learn how you can trust yourself to stick with exercise.

 http://about.com/exercise/committed

| *The* **ABOUT.com** *Guide to* **Getting in Shape**

Chapter 14

Overtraining, Injuries, and Illnesses

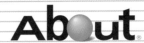

Dealing with Soreness

I remember the first time I ever lifted weights. My sister, a personal trainer at the time, handed me the heaviest pair of dumbbells I'd ever used and took me through one of the hardest upper-body workouts I'd ever done. Looking back now, the workout wasn't that tough, but I wasn't used to lifting challenging weights. I felt good after the workout—until I woke up the next day and realized I was unable to do the simplest of things. Washing my hair was out of the question, since I couldn't lift my arms. To brush my teeth I had to move my head back and forth along the toothbrush, and it was several days before I could function without being in pain.

This was my first real experience with delayed onset muscle soreness (DOMS) and one it took a long time to forget. DOMS isn't unusual after beginning a new exercise program or trying a new activity. In fact, it's likely that most of us will experience some soreness, stiffness, and fatigue within about twelve to forty-eight hours following a new activity. But being sore isn't necessarily an indication of a good workout. You should expect to feel some soreness at first, but if you're consistent with your program, that soreness should go away as your body adapts to what you're doing.

Still, dealing with that level of soreness can be tough, and experts still aren't entirely sure what causes DOMS. Most experts believe that this soreness is caused by microscopic tears in the muscle fibers and that eccentric movements (as opposed to concentric movements) may cause the most soreness. Eccentric contractions are those in which your muscles are contracting as they're lengthening, such as in the lowering phase of a biceps curl or running downhill. But is DOMS inevitable?

It's unlikely that you can completely eliminate soreness from happening; it's something that needs to happen if you want your body to adapt and become stronger and fitter. But being as sore as I was after that first workout and unable to get out of bed means you've probably done too much at one time.

Here are a few steps you can take to avoid getting too sore:

- Warm up before you exercise. This allows your muscles to become more pliable and flexible, which can help them perform better during workouts.
- Stretch after your workouts.
- Ease into new activities. When trying a new cardio workout, start slow and easy and build intensity over time.
- When lifting weights for the first time, stick with one set and choose moderate weights, increasing your intensity over several weeks.

ELSEWHERE ON THE WEB

▶ It's tough to be consistent with exercise, and it becomes tougher if you experience a lot of soreness after that first workout. Realizing that some soreness will probably happen and learning how to handle it will allow you to get back to your workouts, which is what you need to do to keep from getting sore again. About.com's Sports Medicine Guide, Elizabeth Quinn, tells you how to do that in her article "Delayed Onset Muscle Soreness," at http://about.com/sportsmedicine/doms.

- Make small changes to your workouts. Instead of going from ten minutes of walking to forty-five minutes, gradually add a few minutes each week to give your body time to adapt.

Even taking all these precautions, you may end up feeling soreness anyway, and if you overdid it, there are some things you can do to ease the pain a bit. First, you might want to take a few extra recovery days and avoid vigorous exercise, which can make it worse or even cause injury. Taking a hot bath, stretching, icing the sore areas, getting a massage, and taking an OTC anti-inflammatory (such as ibuprofen) can also help deal with the pain. Many exercisers find that light cardio helps increase blood flow to sore muscles, which helps diminish the pain. In my experience, doing a very light version of the workout that made me sore often helps as well. Just make sure you give your body some time to recover before going back to your full routine.

In addition to feeling sore, there are other common aches and pains you might experience when you first start exercising. One of the most common problems is the side stitch, which is often felt by people starting a running program or performing high-impact aerobic activity for the first time. The side stitch feels like a sharp pain near or under the ribcage, and there's no definitive reason why this happens, although some experts believe that the jarring motion of high-impact exercise can cause the ligaments going from the diaphragm to the internal organs to stretch. If you experience a side stitch, stop and walk and try pressing into the area, breathing deeply until it subsides. To prevent side stitches, make sure you don't eat too close to your workout, and breathe deeply and slowly during exercise. Many beginners find that side stitches subside over time as they get into shape.

Another common problem is shin splints, or shooting pains along the front of the leg. Many new walkers and runners experience shin splints when they start exercising, and it can also happen from overdoing it. Some common causes of shin splints include:

- Not warming up before exercise
- Not stretching tight muscles
- Increasing intensity or mileage too quickly
- Wearing worn-out or inappropriate shoes
- Doing high-impact activities on hard surfaces like concrete or asphalt

Elizabeth Quinn, About.com's Sports Medicine Guide, recommends you rest and return to your exercise program gradually. If the pain is intense, you can try RICE (rest, ice, compression, and elevation) to control the swelling, and see your doctor if the problem continues for more than two or three weeks.

Muscle cramps are another common problem you may experience, especially around the calves, hamstrings, quads, and feet. Experts aren't really sure what causes cramps, but they believe that overexertion, inadequate stretching, muscle fatigue, and dehydration can contribute to muscle cramps. Beginners are particularly susceptible because they may experience muscle fatigue more quickly than conditioned exercisers do. To deal with muscle cramps, you can gently stretch and massage the area or apply heat if the area feels tight. To avoid muscle cramps, make sure you're hydrated, that you warm up and stretch, and that you avoid exercising in extreme heat.

Also common to exercisers are pulled or strained muscles. If you don't warm up enough and your muscles are tight, it's possible to overstretch or tear a muscle during a workout or even just doing normal tasks. With a minor strain, you may feel tenderness in the

ELSEWHERE ON THE WEB

▶ Identifying and dealing with the common aches and pains that come with beginning an exercise program can help you stay healthy and feel good during your workouts. About.com's Sports Medicine Guide, Elizabeth Quinn, can help you learn more about your body, how to treat basic injuries, and when it's time to see your doctor. Check out her extensive Pain and Injury Index at http://about.com/sportsmedicine/paininjury.

muscle and limited muscle movement. With a more severe tear, you might have swelling or bruising. With minor strains, you want to avoid aggravating the pain with exercise and follow the same self-care as for other injuries, taking anti-inflammatories or using RICE. If your injury is severe and you can't walk or have a lot of swelling around the injury, you'll want to see your doctor for treatment. You can help prevent muscle strains by warming up before your workouts, stretching tight muscles regularly, and making sure you're getting adequate recovery time between workouts.

Signs of Overtraining

Aches and pains can happen to beginning exercisers, but they can also happen if you overdo it. Too much exercise without enough rest and recovery time can lead to what we call overtraining. Overtraining can make you more susceptible to injuries and illnesses as well as feeling fatigued and out of sorts. Some signs of overtraining include:

- Feeling aches and pains in the muscles and joints
- Trouble sleeping
- Feeling tired or lethargic
- Having an elevated morning pulse
- Feeling depressed
- Being unable to complete your usual workouts
- Loss of appetite
- A decrease in your exercise performance

So, how much is too much exercise? There's no definitive answer to that question since everyone tolerates exercise differently and what's too much for one person may be just fine for another person. The key is to follow a balanced program and exercise for a reasonable period of time, with enough recovery days to

TOOLS YOU NEED

▶ When dealing with swelling, icing the area is a good idea to help reduce inflammation. When the swelling is under control, some heat to the area can ease the discomfort, and it's easier than ever to get relief with the new products available. Try air-activated heat packs that mold to your skin and can be worn under your clothes. There are even pain-relief patches you can apply right to the injured area for instant relief.

▶ If you're sore all the time and can't seem to improve in your workouts, that's one sign you might be doing too much. To learn more about the signs of overtraining, check out my article "Are You Exercising Too Much?" at http://about.com/exercise/toomuch. You'll also find specific tips for dealing with the symptoms of overtraining as well as changes you can make to rest and recover.

allow your body to heal from your workouts. If you do long, intense workouts every day, that kind of schedule could lead to overtraining if you're not careful. By paying attention to how you feel and backing off on days you feel tired, you can keep your workouts at a reasonable level and avoid doing too much. Keeping an exercise journal to track your workouts and how they feel to you is a great tool for keeping your body healthy and rested.

If you do experience these symptoms, you may want to call your doctor first to make sure that nothing else is going on. If it is simply overtraining, your first step is to stop what you're doing and make some changes. If all your workouts are at a high intensity, schedule slower, easier workouts to allow your body to rest and recover. Schedule extra rest days or take several days off from exercise completely. Make sure you're getting enough food to fuel your workouts, since not eating enough calories can make you feel tired and hurt your performance as well as your recovery.

Dealing with Injuries

Having a few aches and pains is one thing, but what if you really hurt yourself? How do you know if you have an injury that needs special treatment or just a passing problem that will heal on its own? There are some general guidelines for when to call your doctor:

- If you experience pain in the joints, especially the knees, ankles, elbows, or wrists.
- If you feel tenderness at a specific place in the body; if you press your fingers into certain places around the bones, muscles, or joints and feel pain, that may be a sign of an injury.
- If you're experiencing swelling or bruising around the injured area.

- If you have reduced range of motion around a joint—swelling in the joint (which isn't visible) may compromise your range of motion.
- Numbness or tingling, which can be a sign of nerve compression.
- Muscle weakness; if a muscle on one side of the body feels significantly weaker than on the other side of the body, that may be a sign of serious injury.

If you ever experience any of these symptoms, stop what you're doing. You should never work through the pain since doing so could make your injury worse. As soon as you identify that something is wrong, you want to start treating it by compressing the area, applying ice to the swelling, elevating the area, and then getting to a doctor for diagnosis or treatment.

The problem with injuries is that, of course, you can't do your normal exercises and you may worry about getting thrown off track or gaining weight. How you handle your injury is important for your mental, as well as physical, well-being. Here are some steps you can take to get through it and take control:

- **Follow doctor's orders.** I've had some clients who decide they're ready for tough workouts before they've gotten clearance. This almost always leads to re-injury, so listen to your doctor.
- **Take control of the situation.** Ask your doctor if there are any exercises you can do without hurting yourself. If you're worried about gaining weight, start looking for ways to reduce your calories if you're going to be inactive for a while.
- **Find creative ways to exercise.** With your doctor's permission, see if there are activities you could do as you wait

ASK YOUR GUIDE

How can I avoid getting injured when I exercise?

▸ Aside from making sure you warm up before exercise and stretch after your workouts, make sure you're wearing supportive shoes. If your shoes are worn out or don't provide the cushioning your body needs, that could lead to injuries. Also, make sure you try new activities from time to time to avoid overuse or repetitive strain injuries. Most of all, get adequate rest between your workouts.

for your injury to heal. If you have a broken arm or injured shoulder, could you do lower-body exercises? If it's a leg injury, could you lift weights for the upper body?

- **Let your body heal.** When you have an injury, that means your body needs to focus energy on healing it. Allow that time, even if it's longer than you want it to be. Going back to exercise too soon could add even more healing time if you hurt yourself all over again.
- **Stay busy.** Some exercisers get depressed when they get injured or sick. Instead, use the time you have to focus on other things, like catching up on your reading or spending time with your family. Making the best of your healing time will make it go much faster.

Should You Exercise When You're Sick?

Even more common than injuries are those random illnesses that seem to hit when you don't have time to be sick. Most of us occasionally catch a cold or the flu or experience sinus infections, bronchitis, or other illnesses, and it's hard to know if exercise will make you feel better or if it will only make things worse. Most experts suggest that if your symptoms are above the neck (e.g., sniffles and a runny nose), you can probably exercise, although you may want to lower the intensity of your workouts. If your workout makes you feel worse, that's a sign your body may need some rest, so take it easy. You should skip your workouts if you:

- **Have a fever and/or body aches and pains.** This often means you're fighting an infection and exercising can make it worse.

- **Have a persistent cough.** This may mean you have an upper respiratory infection of some kind and your lung capacity may be diminished.
- **Are nauseated or have diarrhea.** If you're fighting stomach problems, your body may be dehydrated and exercise can only make it worse.
- **Have a serious illness or condition.** If you have the flu, pneumonia, or bronchitis, follow your doctor's orders and don't exercise until you get medical clearance.

If you have a serious illness, you probably aren't jazzed about working out anyway, but what about other problems like hangovers or jet lag? If you have a hangover, one reason you feel so bad is that you're dehydrated. I have many clients who think they can "sweat out" the pain, but that isn't a good idea since exercise can only exacerbate the problem. The same is true of jet lag if you haven't been getting enough water. So, wait until you've rehydrated, and if you decide to exercise, lower the intensity of your workout.

Another problem some exercisers may experience is exercise-induced asthma. Asthma happens when the breathing passages of the lungs become inflamed, making it difficult to breathe. Some people may have no problems with asthma until they start exercising, and one reason is a change in the temperature and humidity of the air you're breathing. Because you usually breathe through your mouth when you exercise, the air you're breathing is colder and drier when it hits the lungs, which may trigger an attack. Experts believe that exercising in cold temperatures or doing activities that require short bursts of speed (like football or handball) can often trigger exercise-induced asthma in people sensitive to it.

If you've never had experience with asthma, you may not be familiar with the symptoms; they can include wheezing, coughing, tightness in the chest, and fatigue. The good news is that exercise-induced asthma can be treated so that you can continue exercising without discomfort. Your first step is, of course, to see your doctor for diagnosis. He or she may prescribe an inhaler you can use before you exercise, to prevent an attack. Your doctor may also recommend avoiding exercise in cold weather and on days with a high pollen count if you have allergies or if you have any other respiratory problems from a cold or the flu.

If you do get sick or become injured, getting back to your usual workouts can feel overwhelming. If you've taken several days or weeks off from exercise, your body has certainly lost some of the muscle strength and cardio endurance you've been building. One mistake many people make is trying to go back to the schedule they were following before the injury or illness. This is a bad idea. Not only could you re-injure yourself by doing too much too soon, but you may feel discouraged if you can't make it through the workout.

To make the transition easier, start with a light program and gradually add intensity as your body gets stronger. You may need more rest days to recover, and you also may need to cut the intensity of your workouts for several days or weeks until you gain strength. If you're recovering from an injury, you may need to perform exercises prescribed by a physical therapist before getting back to your normal strength-training routine. If that's the case, do it! I've had many clients healing from knee or back injuries who stop doing physical therapy exercises because they're bored or they start to feel better and think they don't need them anymore. Inevitably, this often leads to re-injury or chronic problems that take even longer to heal. It may take a while to heal an injury, but following your doctor's orders and giving your body the time it needs may save you time in the end and leave you with a stronger foundation to work from.

Get Linked

The following resources at my **About.com** *Exercise site provide more insight into dealing with injuries, illnesses, overtraining, and burnout. By recognizing when you need to change what you're doing, take a break, or ease off, you can keep your body and mind strong for the long haul.*

HEALING MOVES

Exercise can often be used to manage common ailments like arthritis, depression, and heart disease, and authors Carol and Mitchell Krucoff describe ways to get more out of your life in their book, *Healing Moves*. Check out my review to find out more.

 http://about.com/exercise/healingmoves

10 WAYS YOU KNOW YOU'RE BURNED OUT ON EXERCISE

This article offers a humorous take on burnout, describing a few symptoms you may experience when your routine is getting stale, along with some tips for shaking things up.

 http://about.com/exercise/burnedout

GETTING THROUGH AN INJURY OR ILLNESS

Allowing your body time to get over an injury or illness can be a tough mental challenge. One way to handle it is to take control and be involved in your own healing process. This article offers more in-depth tips for what you can do to speed the healing process.

 http://about.com/exercise/injuryillness

The **ABOUT.com** *Guide to* **Getting in Shape**

Chapter 15

Special Situations

Pregnancy

I've worked with a number of pregnant clients over the years, and they all agree that exercise makes pregnancy easier, labor and delivery better, and postpartum weight loss much faster. In fact, the American College of Sports Medicine recently released a statement saying that exercise during pregnancy can reduce the risk of preeclampsia, can help manage gestational diabetes, can alleviate pregnancy-related aches and pains, and helps improve your mood and energy level. They also found that exercise while breastfeeding doesn't effect milk production or infant growth.

If you've been exercising regularly before pregnancy, you should be able to maintain your program to some degree throughout your pregnancy, unless your doctor tells you otherwise. Some women are afraid that exercise can cause miscarriages, but there's no evidence of that if you follow a safe program. The key is to adjust your program throughout your pregnancy and focus on maintaining

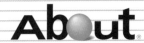

Is it safe to exercise during pregnancy?

▶ For healthy women with normal pregnancies, exercise can be very safe. Your doctor may restrict your exercise if you've had pre-term labor or problems with previous pregnancies, so you should always get clearance from your doctor. But if you have no restrictions, following a balanced program that targets strength, endurance, and flexibility can keep you healthy and strong throughout your pregnancy.

your strength and fitness in a way that fits with how you feel and with how your body is changing.

If you're pregnant and you've never exercised, now isn't the time to decide you want to run a marathon, become a powerlifter, or lose some weight. But you can safely start an exercise program if you take some precautions. The American College of Obstetricians and Gynecologists has posted guidelines for exercising during pregnancy and suggests:

- Pregnant women who are healthy should do thirty minutes of moderate exercise on most days of the week (with a doctor's clearance, of course).
- Avoid lying on your back after the first trimester since this can reduce blood flow to the womb.
- Most activities are fine during pregnancy, but avoid exercises with a high risk of falling or abdominal trauma, like horseback riding, skiing, and soccer.
- Stop exercising and see your doctor if you have any bleeding, dizziness, headaches, chest pains, muscle weakness, or signs of preterm labor.

So, what type of exercise should you do when you're pregnant? In general, the same exercises anyone should do: cardio exercise, strength training, and yoga or flexibility exercises. The difference is that your focus is on being healthy and strong throughout your pregnancy and during labor and delivery rather than building endurance or losing weight. Two favorite cardio activities for pregnant women are walking and swimming. Both of these can keep your heart strong and can help you feel comfortable as your center of gravity changes throughout your pregnancy.

What you do will often depend on where you are in your pregnancy. During the first trimester, you may experience morning sickness and fatigue, so you may not exercise as much as you'd like. When you're feeling better, you can start with a light cardio program at a moderate intensity. Just be sure to listen to your body and don't overexert yourself or exercise in extreme temperatures.

Strength training is also important during pregnancy, but you do want to take some precautions. Experts recommend you use slow, controlled movements and lighter weights to prevent injuries caused by loosened joints. They also recommend avoiding standing exercises during your second and third trimester, which can cause dizziness as the blood pools in your legs. If you decide to strength train during pregnancy, stick with a simple, basic program with moves that target the entire body and use moderate weights. There are a number of exercise videos targeting pregnant women, and they offer safe, effective workouts you can do throughout your pregnancy to remain strong and fit. Check out CollageVideo.com (http://collagevideo.com) for some ideas.

Many women find that yoga is a great choice during pregnancy. It's relaxing and soothing, and at the same time you're building strength and flexibility. It can also be a good choice on those days when you're too tired for more intense workouts. In addition, the focus on deep breathing can help you learn to relax and can benefit you during labor and delivery. Some precautions to take when doing yoga include:

- Avoid poses that stretch the body too much; your body releases a hormone during pregnancy that relaxes the joints and connective tissue, so it's easier to tear or strain muscles when you're pregnant.
- Use a chair or wall for support during balancing poses.
- Avoid postures that have you lying on your back during the second and third trimesters.

ELSEWHERE ON THE WEB

▸ Exercise can be a great tool for managing stress and keeping the body strong during pregnancy. To learn more about how you can incorporate exercise safely into your life, check out the article "Pregnancy Fitness and Exercise" by About.com's Pregnancy Guide, Robin Elise Weiss. Here you'll find specific tips for how to safely begin an exercise program wherever you are in your pregnancy (http://about.com/pregnancy/pregfitness).

- Avoid moves that strain or compress the belly and inverted poses like headstands or shoulder stands.
- Listen to your body and skip any moves that make you nervous or make you feel that you'll lose your balance.

If you're experienced with yoga, you may be able to modify the poses on your own to fit where you are in your pregnancy. If you're taking a class, talk with the instructor to get specific modifications or take a yoga class specifically created for pregnancy. If you're new to yoga, you might try a video or book to help you learn safe yoga postures during pregnancy.

Above all, make sure you listen to your body and do what you can. You may find your energy levels changing wildly from trimester to trimester—perhaps even from day to day—and you may need to be flexible about your exercise.

After you've had the baby and are ready to get back to exercise, you'll need to get clearance from your doctor to start your workouts. If you've been exercising all through your pregnancy, you may find you can start light activity within a few days after giving birth, if you had a normal vaginal delivery. If you've had a C-section, it may be six weeks or more before you can safely start exercising. Again, your doctor will be able to help you determine the right time to start exercising.

Obesity

If you're overweight or obese, you probably already know that exercise is a good idea for managing your weight. But you may also find it's difficult to do physical activities and that traditional exercise may not always work for you. I recently worked with two obese clients and one thing we discovered right away was that we would have to be creative with their workouts. Not only did they have problems fitting on the machines, but many exercises

▶ If you're interested in trying yoga, you'll want yoga workouts specifically for different stages of pregnancy. There are some postures you may need to avoid depending on how far along you are, and you may not always know how to modify typical workouts to make them safe. Sara Holliday's *Prenatal Yoga* DVD is perfect for women in their first trimester, providing a safe, effective yoga workout. Check out my review at http://about.com/exercise/prenatalyoga.

were impossible for them to do. Squats were difficult because of knee and ankle problems, getting up and down from the floor was something both women struggled with, and it was often a matter of trial and error finding activities they could do without pain or difficulty. But putting our heads together, we managed to come up with an exercise program that worked for them, and one reason was because they were willing to keep trying.

Unfortunately, for every obese client who finds the courage to start an exercise program, there are hundreds of others who are so intimidated by the thought of exercise, they don't even want to try. Joining a gym is often out of the question—what if you can't fit on the machines? How will you make it through an entire workout if you have low endurance and strength? What will all those skinny people think of you? Not only that, but there are a number of physical problems you may experience, such as:

- Balance problems
- Muscle weakness
- Aches and pains in the joints and lower back
- Difficulty moving
- Poor circulation
- Muscle cramps
- Chafing

There are a number of obstacles you may have to overcome if you're obese and beginning an exercise program, but the good news is, just getting started with any kind of activity will put you on the right track, and you don't have to join a gym to do it.

Before you start any kind of exercise program, always see your doctor to make sure you're on top of any other medical issues you may have, such as hypertension, diabetes, or heart problems. Once you do that, you may want to consider a few options for starting an

▶ It's hard to find exercise equipment to fit larger people comfortably, but one piece of equipment on the market is the NuStep TRS 4000 (www.nustep.com). It's a recumbent cross trainer and is designed to fit every body type and size while reducing stress on the joints. This cardio exercise involves both the upper and lower body for a low-impact full-body workout.

exercise program. First, consider hiring a personal trainer either at a studio or in your own home. You'll have privacy and access to an expert to help you set up a safe, effective program where you can focus your attention on building strength, endurance, and more functionality. If that isn't an option, there are some things you can do at home to get in shape.

One option is to use home fitness equipment, and a great choice for low-impact, supportive exercise is a recumbent bike. If you have joint problems or lower-back pain, a recumbent bike can provide extra support for your body during cardio exercise. If you have limited space or a limited budget, you can consider portable equipment such as cycle machines that can be used for the arms or the legs. This type of equipment is usually less expensive and can often be used while in a seated position if mobility is an issue (check out ComfortChannel.com for ideas).

Walking is always a great choice because you can do it anywhere and you don't need any special equipment. You can even do all your walking inside if that's more comfortable for you, and there are a number of videos, such as those offered by Leslie Sansone (www.lesliesansone.com), that provide walking workouts you can do in the comfort of your own living room. You can also try other types of videos, such as the Sit and Be Fit series (www.sitandbefit .com).

Another great tool is a pedometer, which keeps track of your steps each day. By recording how many steps you take, you can set goals to increase those steps until you're up to at least 10,000, which is equivalent to about thirty minutes of moderate exercise a day, as recommended by the surgeon general.

You can also practice more functional training if you have problems with mobility or regular daily activities. Standing up and sitting down is something many overweight people struggle with. One of my obese clients told me her goal was to be able to get up from a chair without moaning and groaning. To reach her goal, we had her practice sitting and standing, first using the back of a chair to give her leverage and then taking that away so she had to use her own strength. Try it yourself several times throughout the day and you'll notice an improvement.

Another common problem is getting up and down stairs or stepping up onto curbs and keeping your balance. You can practice this by standing in front of a stair or step and just tapping the top of the step with your toes, alternating feet. You can hold on to a wall or a chair for balance and gradually take your hand away so you're balancing on your own. Once you've mastered that, step up onto the step with the right foot, bringing the left foot up as well and then step down, practicing on both feet. This is also a great cardio exercise if you continue stepping for several minutes. Just make sure there's a handrail nearby in case you need it.

One obese client told me he wanted to be able to get in and out of his car without embarrassing himself. Part of our weekly workout involved him sitting in his car and learning to position himself so he could get out more easily. We also used resistance bands and dumbbells to build up his arm and leg strength so he could push or pull himself out with a minimum of fuss. His weight loss was gradual, but just being able to function better motivated him to continue working out on a regular basis.

The key is to find any activity, whether it's walking down to the mailbox or just walking around your house, and map out a plan to do it every day. Pick up some dumbbells or even full cans of soup if you don't have weights and do some biceps curls or overhead presses. Set goals to exercise for a certain amount of time each day, and improve on that each week by adding a few minutes at a time. Most of all, talk to your doctor and find out about any resources that might be available to you through a hospital gym, nutritionist, or personal trainer. Some areas have programs that help obese and

TOOLS YOU NEED

▶ If you're overweight or obese and have a hard time moving around, it may seem impossible to get any exercise in. Even if you have to remain seated, you can always get some type of exercise in and that can help you progress to more intense exercise. This Seated Total Body Strength Workout (http://about.com/exercise/seatedtotalbody) offers strength-training moves that target the upper and lower body and are perfect for seated exercise.

overweight people tackle their weight problems in all areas, from fitness to food issues.

Seniors and Exercise

These days it may seem like aging gracefully is more about plastic surgery than anything else. But no amount of plastic surgery can stop our bodies from getting older. What we can control is how we age and how healthy and strong we are as we get older. Regular exercise, including cardio, strength training, and flexibility training can keep you agile, flexible, and mobile throughout your life.

If you don't exercise on a regular basis as you get older, you may find certain areas of fitness and health diminishing. For example, you may experience:

- **Loss of muscle mass.** Some experts suggest we can lose up to 4 percent of muscle each decade after the age of twenty-five if we don't lift weights. That loss of muscle also means loss of strength and a slower metabolism.
- **Loss of endurance.** If you don't do regular cardio exercise, you may also lose cardio endurance as you age, which can lead to decreased mobility.
- **Loss of balance.** This is one common problem seen in older adults if they don't exercise and work on their balance on a regular basis. Broken hips are a common problem with seniors and will often cause them to be more cautious when moving around, which can compromise flexibility and mobility.
- **Loss of flexibility.** If you don't regularly stretch your muscles, they may become tighter as you get older, which is another cause of balance problems, falling, and just being less functional in life.

The National Institute on Aging believes that one reason we experience so many health problems as we age isn't just because we're getting older, it's because we've become inactive. Luckily, these kinds of health issues can be prevented with a complete exercise program, and even if you've never followed a structured exercise routine, it's never too late to start.

The first step to better health as you age is to, of course, get moving by incorporating cardio, strength training, and flexibility training into your daily life. If you haven't exercised in a long time or are under a doctor's care for any reason, you should get clearance from your doctor before you start exercising. If you have special situations like arthritis, osteoporosis, diabetes, heart disease, or other conditions, you may need to make some modifications to your program.

Once you get cleared for exercise, you'll want to set up a simple program that incorporates each element of fitness. If you've never lifted weights, you may think it's too late if you're an older adult. But you don't have to lift massive weights or follow a hardcore routine to get the benefit of weight training. In fact, you could set up a simple program with a few basic exercises with moderate weight and see significant improvements in your coordination, balance, and strength in short, simple workouts.

The following are a few basic guidelines to follow:

- Lift weights at least twice a week for the major muscle groups of the body; a typical full-body workout might include chair squats, leg lifts, leg extensions, chest presses, seated rows, lateral raises, biceps curls, triceps extensions, abdominal crunches, and back extensions.
- Start with no weights or very light weights to practice your form; you may want to start with machines and move on to free weights when you've mastered those.

- Start with one set of about fifteen repetitions of each exercise and eventually work your way up to a weight you can lift only fifteen times.
- To progress, add a set after a few weeks of regular strength training.

For cardio exercise, any activity you enjoy and that feels good to you will work. Walking is a favorite choice for seniors as are water aerobics, cycling, and aerobics or jazzercise classes. If you haven't done any cardio in a while, give your body some time to build endurance. You may want to start with a few minutes a day and gradually add on to that each week until you're up to thirty or more minutes.

Last, you'll want to incorporate some flexibility exercises into your routine if you haven't already done so. When stretching, you want to make sure your muscles are warm (such as after a walk or a hot shower), and you also want to focus on stretching different areas of your body for better mobility, range of motion, and daily functioning. Some stretches you can try include:

- **Hamstring stretch.** To stretch this muscle, you can sit on a chair and take the right leg straight out in front with the foot flexed. Gently lean forward, keeping the back flat, until you feel a stretch in the back of the leg. Hold for fifteen to thirty seconds and repeat on the other leg.
- **Hips and quads.** Hold onto a chair for balance and take the right leg back in a split stance. Bend the knees and lower into a slight lunge, gently squeezing the glutes and pressing the right hip forward to stretch the front of the leg. Hold for fifteen to thirty seconds and switch legs.
- **Calves.** Stand on a step or raised surface and take the right heel back off the step, gently pressing down to feel

ELSEWHERE ON THE WEB

▶ If you're interested in starting a cardio program, you'll want to make sure you start slowly and set up a safe routine that fits your fitness level. For details about different activities you can do, About.com's Senior Living Guide, Sharon O'Brien, offers tips in her article "Cardio Exercises for a Healthy Heart," at http://about.com/seniorliving/cardioheart. You'll also find details for how often to exercise and for keeping your workouts comfortable and safe.

a stretch in the calf. Hold for fifteen to thirty seconds and switch legs.

- **Hips and glutes.** Lie on the floor with the knees bent and bring the right knee in to the chest, holding it just behind the knee (you can straighten the left leg for a deeper stretch). Hold for fifteen to thirty seconds and switch legs.

Kids and Teens

Another population fitness and health experts are focusing on these days is kids. Most of us are aware that many kids are overweight and some are experiencing health problems that only adults previously experienced, like heart disease and type 2 diabetes. Trying to get ourselves to exercise is hard enough; trying to get kids to exercise can be even harder, especially if their schools don't include a fitness or PE program but have plenty of fast food and soda to go around. Despite the difficulties, getting kids to be more active is essential, for both their physical health and mental health. Some of the problems overweight kids face include:

- Depression and low self-esteem
- Aches and pains in the bones and joints
- Increased risk of type 2 diabetes
- Increased risk of heart disease
- A higher likelihood of being overweight or obese as an adult

The reasons kids are overweight are often the same reasons adults are: poor diet, lack of exercise, genetics, and too much time involved in sedentary activities. So, if that's the case, how can you get your child to exercise, and what should he or she be doing?

▶ Yoga is an excellent choice if you want to start exercising but want something gentle that will improve your balance, strength, and flexibility. If you're new to yoga or any type of exercise, you'll want to start with a beginner class or video. There are also yoga videos available just for seniors, such as *Yoga for the Young at Heart*, at Yogaheart .com.

What do you do if you're worried your child might be overweight?

▶ If your child is overweight, you may not know how to deal with it or where to start, especially if you're struggling with your own weight problems. For specifics on what causes childhood obesity and tips for creating a healthy environment, check out my article "Understanding and Dealing with Childhood Obesity," at http:// about.com/exercise/child obesity. You'll also find ideas for getting your kids to exercise more.

Your first step is doing what you can to change the environment so that your child is surrounded by a healthier atmosphere. That often means changing your own behavior as well because you are your child's most important role model, and he or she will see what you do and learn from that.

Part of this is teaching your child how to eat in healthy ways. It can be a chore to wean kids off of sweets and junk food, but if this type of thing isn't in the house in the first place, the entire family will find it easier to avoid too much junk. Many experts suggest getting your kids involved in both the shopping and the cooking so that they can help make decisions regarding what they eat. Remember that being healthy doesn't mean you have to get rid of all junk food forever, but moderate it and allow it to be a treat rather than something children have every day.

For exercise, the focus should be on being more active and having fun rather than putting kids on a rigid exercise routine (unless that's something they would enjoy). One way many parents get their kids to exercise is to plan fun family activities like playing in the park, riding bikes around the neighborhood, or tossing a ball in the backyard. By getting involved, you'll get some exercise in too, and your kids will learn that moving around can be fun.

For things your child can do on his own, choose activities that fit your child's personality. If he doesn't like team sports, signing him up for basketball or soccer may not be a good idea—but he might enjoy riding his bike with you on your walk. If your daughter loves turning flips and tumbling around the house, you might consider a gymnastics program. Other ideas to consider include swimming, martial arts, dancing, surfing, snowboarding, and inline skating. Just make sure you and your child work together to find ways she can be active while having fun so she'll keep exercising for the long term.

Strength training is also an option for kids and teens and is becoming increasingly popular, especially in fitness classes in many schools. Though some people still believe that strength training can stunt growth in kids, there's no evidence of that if kids are following a safe program. The biggest concern is preventing injuries, which can happen if kids lift too much weight or don't use good form, a common problem if they don't have a coach or other expert supervising. In fact, strength training can have a number of benefits for kids, including:

- A better attitude toward being active and fit
- Improved strength and endurance
- Increase in bone density
- Enhanced coordination and body composition
- Reduced risk of injury

In general, if your child is old enough to participate in organized sports (about seven or eight), he or she can probably handle a basic strength-training program. Your child should be coordinated enough to perform the exercise and should be able to follow directions to do the moves correctly. To make sure your kids lift weight safely, make sure they're supervised and know how to use good form for the exercises. In general, most kids can start with about six to eight exercises and perform one set of fifteen reps using light to medium weights. As they become stronger, they can increase the weight gradually and add more exercises. Most of all, they should be having fun, so consider a variety of tools and toys like medicine balls, resistance tubes, and other equipment they might have fun learning to use.

ELSEWHERE ON THE WEB

▶ It may be tough to tear your kids away from the computer or the TV for exercise—unless, of course, it's something that sounds fun to them. If they have fun with exercise, it's something they'll keep doing, and they'll be less likely to have health and weight problems when they get older. To learn more about how to get your kids excited about exercise, check out the article "Kids and Exercise" at www.kidshealth.org/parent/nutrition_fit/fitness/exercise.html.

Get Linked

The following resources at my About.com *Exercise site provide more information about how to deal with special situations such as pregnancy, senior fitness, and exercise for kids.*

EXERCISING DURING PREGNANCY

This article offers detailed information for how to start an exercise program when you're pregnant. Also included are resources for finding comfortable maternity clothes and free walking programs.

 http://about.com/exercise/pregexercise

TOTAL BODY STRENGTH FOR SENIORS

I've worked with a number of older adults and most of them have a hard time picturing themselves lifting weights, especially if they've never tried it before. This workout offers some simple exercises anyone can do with very little equipment.

 http://about.com/exercise/totalbodysenior

TEENAGERS AND EXERCISE

More and more teens are starting to lift weights, and for most teens, that's a good thing. But there are some precautions teens should take when it comes to resistance training, and this article offers some dos and don'ts for safe exercise.

 http://about.com/exercise/teenagers

Appendix A

Glossary

abduct
> The movement of lifting a limb away from the midline of the body.

active isolated stretching (AIS)
> A type of stretching in which you actively contract the muscle opposite the target muscle.

adduction
> The movement of drawing a limb toward the midline of the body.

aerobic
> When exercising aerobically, you're improving oxygen consumption by the body.

anaerobic
> When exercising anaerobically, you're doing an activity in which the body incurs an oxygen debt.

basal metabolic rate (BMR)
> The minimum amount of energy your body needs to sustain basic and vital functions or the energy expended by your body at rest to maintain normal function.

bioelectrical impedance analysis (BIA)
A type of body-fat monitoring system in which a low-level electrical signal is sent through the body to measure body composition.

body composition
The ratio or percentage of body fat to lean muscle tissue.

body fat percentage
The percentage of your body made up of fatty tissue.

body mass index (BMI)
A measurement of whether you're overweight or underweight, derived from a formula using body weight and height.

calipers
A measuring device used to measure body fat at different points of the body to determine body fat percentage.

compound movements
Exercises that involve more than one muscle group and more than one joint movement at the same time.

concentric
A contraction in which the muscle shortens and exerts force to overcome resistance.

cross-training
A method of training in which a variety of exercises are used to work the body in different ways, to increase motivation and protect the body from repetitive strain injuries.

delayed onset muscle soreness (DOMS)
Muscle soreness that occurs twenty-four to forty-eight hours after exercise, due to microscopic tears in the muscle fibers.

DEXA
A whole-body scanner used to determine body fat and bone density.

eccentric
A contraction in which the muscle lengthens as it contracts.

elevation
The act of lifting or raising the shoulder blades.

extension
A movement at a joint that brings two bones into a straight line, which increases the angle at the joint.

fast-twitch muscle fibers
A type of muscle fiber that is characterized by its speed of contraction and used during explosive, anaerobic movements.

flexion
A movement at the joint in which the bones are brought closer together.

heart rate reserve (HRR)
The result of subtracting resting heart rate from maximum heart rate.

hydrostatic weighing
 A method for measuring lean body mass in which a person is weighed underwater.

hypertrophy
 An increase in the size of the muscles.

interval training
 A type of training in which you alternate short, high-intensity exercise with lower-intensity periods of rest.

maximum heart rate (MHR)
 The highest heart rate a person can attain.

nutrient dense
 A type of food that provides more nutrients per calorie.

one rep maximum (I RM)
 The amount of weight a muscle can lift one time to fatigue.

overtraining
 Intense training that does not provide adequate rest and recovery for the body, leading to decreased performance, elevated resting heart rate, and decreased enthusiasm for exercise.

periodization
 A systematic plan in which you vary different elements of your program to optimize results.

plyometric exercises
    Explosive movements that teach the muscles to produce maximum force faster.

pyramid training
    A method of strength training in which you increase the weight and decrease the number of reps (or vice versa) during each set.

range of motion
    How far a muscle can flex and extend.

rate of perceived exertion (RPE)
    A scale that provides a way to measure how hard an exercise feels.

resting heart rate (RHR)
    The number of times the heart beats per minute when the body is at rest.

retraction
    The act of adducting the shoulder blades, or bringing them closer together.

rotation
    The act of turning a body part around a center or an axis.

slow-twitch muscle fibers
    A type of muscle characterized by its slow speed of contraction, used during endurance activities.

supersets
　　A method of strength training in which you perform two or more exercises for the same muscle group consecutively.

supination
　　A joint movement that includes dorsiflexion, adduction, and inversion, as when you turn your arm so that the palm faces forward.

target heart rate zone
　　The number of heart beats associated with the most efficient level of intensity for cardio exercise.

thermic effect of food (TEF)
　　Energy that is expended when food is digested.

tri-sets
　　A method of strength training in which you perform three exercises for the same muscle group consecutively.

waist-hip ratio
　　A measure that divides the waist measurement by the hip measurement to determine health risks.

Appendix B

Other Sites

About.com Bodybuilding

You don't have to be a bodybuilder to appreciate Hugo Rivera's site. He offers great information about building muscle, losing fat, and beginning a strength-training program.

http://bodybuilding.about.com

About.com Nutrition

Shereen Jegtvig's Nutrition site offers a wealth of information about the basics of nutrition. Here you'll find information about low-carb diets, essential nutrients your body needs, healthy recipes, and more.

http://nutrition.about.com

About.com Running/Jogging

Whether you want to run a marathon or just make it around the block, Jesslyn Cummings can help you figure out where to start, with articles, step-by-step guides, shoe reviews, and free running programs.

http://running.about.com

About.com Pilates

Marguerite Ogle's Pilates site provides detailed information about Pilates. You'll learn about the principles behind Pilates, how to breathe during Pilates exercises, how to find a good teacher, and basic Pilates exercises.

http://pilates.about.com

About.com Pregnancy/Birth

If you're interested in learning more about how to have a healthy pregnancy as well as what you can expect at every point of your pregnancy, visit Robin Elise Weiss's Pregnancy site. She offers articles and tips for getting pregnant, prenatal health, postpartum issues, and more.

http://pregnancy.about.com

About.com Sports Medicine

Whether you're a full-time athlete or a weekend warrior, you'll find great information at Elizabeth Quinn's Sports Medicine site. She covers the ins and outs of sports injuries, the basics of strength training, and how to get the most out of your body no matter what activities you're involved in.

http://sportsmedicine.about.com

About.com Walking

Wendy Bumgardner's Walking site should be your first stop if you'd like to start a walking program. She has a number of free walking programs and workouts as well as information about tools, clothing, shoes, and more.

http://walking.about.com

About.com Weight Loss

Jennifer R. Scott's Weight Loss site offers great information about losing weight, including tips for beginners, detailed articles about specific diets, and information on exercise.

http://weightloss.about.com

About.com Yoga

If you'd like to learn more about yoga, especially how to do a variety of yoga postures, visit Ann Pizer's site. She has an extensive database and photo gallery of yoga poses as well as great information about how to get started and which type of yoga is best for you.

http://yoga.about.com

American Council on Exercise Library

If you're looking for new and interesting exercise ideas, ACE offers an extensive library that includes everything from balance and stability moves to yoga and strength-training exercises.

www.acefitness.org/getfit/freeexercise.aspx

Calorie Control Council

This site offers information about cutting calories in your diet to lose weight and get healthy. There are a variety of tools like calorie and activity calculators as well as a wealth of recipes and articles about eating healthy.

www.caloriecontrol.org

ExRx.net

This site offers a wealth of information about exercise, fitness, and nutrition. It has an extensive database of exercises as well as information about exercise guidelines, strength training, cardio exercise, and more.

www.exrx.net

Plus One Active

Plus One Active offers a variety of online personal training programs. You can choose to work with a trainer and receive a variety of workouts, or if you're more independent, you can sign up to receive a workout program without access to a trainer.

www.plusoneactive.com

Workouts for Women

This site offers online personal training programs for women as well as advice on nutrition, weight loss, and fitness.

www.workoutsforwomen.com

Appendix C

Further Reading

The Athletic-Minded Traveler **by Jim Kaese and Paul Huddle**

This is an excellent resource for travelers. This book offers descriptions of hundreds of different hotels in major cities, with a specific focus on fitness. You'll get expert advice on where to stay for the best fitness facilities; walking, jogging and bike paths; and more.

Body for Life **by Bill Phillips**

Bill Phillips offers a twelve-week program that includes cardio and strength training as well as nutritional and motivational advice for getting fit and losing weight.

Body for Life for Women **by Pam Peeke**

This is an excellent resource for women in all stages of fitness and in life. Dr. Peeke offers a strength-training and cardio program for fitness and weight loss as well as excellent advice for how the body changes in different stages of life.

The Complete Idiot's Guide to Weight Loss **by Lucy Beale and Sandy G. Couvillon**

Authors Lucy Beale and Sandy G. Couvillon offer a healthy way to lose weight without living on "lettuce and carrot juice," as they put it. The book includes weight loss and nutritional plans; information on carbs, protein, and fat; as well as alternative approaches to dieting.

Eating Thin for Life: Food Secrets & Recipes from People Who Have Lost Weight & Kept It Off by Anne M. Fletcher

> The best advice you can get is sometimes from real people who've managed to lose weight and keep it off. This book offers the experiences of over 200 people who have created and maintained healthy lifestyles.

Encyclopedia of Muscle & Strength by Jim Stoppani

> This research-based book gets a little technical, but if you want to truly understand the principles behind building muscle and strength as well as have an in-depth look at the muscles and what they do, this book is a great resource. It also includes exercises and workout programs designed to build mass and strength.

Getting in Shape by Bob Anderson, Bill Pearl, and Ed Burke

> This short but well-constructed book takes you through the basics of getting in shape. The first part of the book includes thirty-two different exercise programs that include cardio, strength, and flexibility exercises. The second part covers the principles of exercise as well as healthy eating, weight loss, exercising with health conditions, and more.

Strength Training Past 50 by Wayne L. Westcott and Thomas R. Baechle

> This book is a great resource for exercisers in their fifties and older. The authors discuss the reasons that strength training is so important, especially for seniors, and offers strength tests as well as programs to increase strength and endurance.

YOU: The Owner's Manual by Michael F. Roizen and Mehmet Oz

This easy-to-read book covers every part of the human body, from how your thyroid works to basic anatomy and physiology of the human body. It also includes a food plan and guidelines for a basic exercise program.

INDEX

▶ IT'S **About**® *INFORMATION DELIVERED IN A REVOLUTIONARY NEW WAY.*

The Internet. Books. Experts. This is how—and where—we get our information today. And now, the best of these resources are available together in a revolutionary new series of how-to guides from **About.com** and Adams Media.

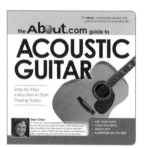

The About.com Guide to Acoustic Guitar
ISBN 10: 1-59869-098-1
ISBN 13: 978-1-59869-098-9

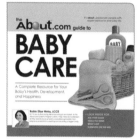

The About.com Guide to Baby Care
ISBN 10: 1-59869-274-7
ISBN 13: 978-1-59869-274-7

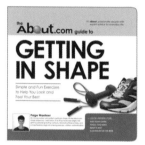

The About.com Guide to Getting in Shape
ISBN 10: 1-59869-278-X
ISBN 13: 978-1-59869-278-5

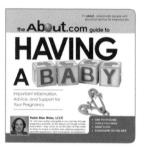

The About.com Guide to Having a Baby
ISBN 10: 1-59869-095-7
ISBN 13: 978-1-59869-095-8

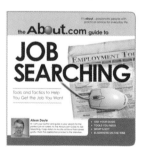

The About.com Guide to Job Searching
ISBN 10: 1-59869-097-3
ISBN 13: 978-1-59869-097-2

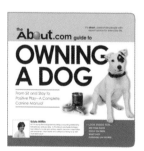

The About.com Guide to Owning a Dog
ISBN 10: 1-59869-279-8
ISBN 13: 978-1-59869-279-2

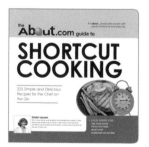

The About.com Guide to Shortcut Cooking
ISBN 10: 1-59869-273-9
ISBN 13: 978-1-59869-273-0

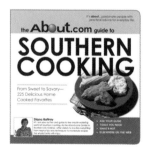

The About.com Guide to Southern Cooking
ISBN 10: 1-59869-096-5
ISBN 13: 978-1-59869-096-5

Available wherever books are sold! Or call us at 1-800-258-0929 or visit us at *www.adamsmedia.com.*